Treatment Manual for Smoking Cessation Groups
A Guide for Therapists

Treatment Manual for Smoking Cessation Groups

A Guide for Therapists

Werner G. K. Stritzke

Joyce L. Y. Chong

Diane Ferguson

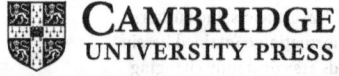
CAMBRIDGE
UNIVERSITY PRESS

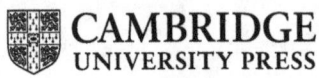

Shaftesbury Road, Cambridge CB2 8EA, United Kingdom

One Liberty Plaza, 20th Floor, New York, NY 10006, USA

477 Williamstown Road, Port Melbourne, VIC 3207, Australia

314–321, 3rd Floor, Plot 3, Splendor Forum, Jasola District Centre, New Delhi – 110025, India

103 Penang Road, #05–06/07, Visioncrest Commercial, Singapore 238467

Cambridge University Press is part of Cambridge University Press & Assessment,
a department of the University of Cambridge.

We share the University's mission to contribute to society through the pursuit of
education, learning and research at the highest international levels of excellence.

www.cambridge.org
Information on this title: www.cambridge.org/9780521709255

First published 2009

A catalogue record for this publication is available from the British Library

Library of Congress Cataloging-in-Publication data
Stritzke, Werner G. K., 1956–
     Treatment manual for smoking cessation groups : a guide for therapists / Werner G.K. Stritzke,
Joyce L.Y. Chong, Diane Ferguson.
          p.   ;   cm.
     Includes bibliographical references and index.
     ISBN 978-0-521-70925-5 (paperback)
1. Smoking cessation–Handbooks, manuals, etc.   2. Group psychotherapy–Handbooks, manuals, etc.
I. Chong, Joyce L. Y.   II. Ferguson, Diane, 1977–   III. Title.
[DNLM: 1. Smoking Cessation–methods.   2. Smoking Cessation–psychology.   3. Psychotherapy, Group–
methods.   WM 290 S918t 2009]
     RC567.S82 2009
     616.86'506–dc22

                                                                                        2008029665

ISBN   978-0-521-70925-5   Paperback

....

Every effort has been made in preparing this book to provide accurate and up-to-date
information which is in accord with accepted standards and practice at the time of
publication. Although case histories are drawn from actual cases, every effort has been
made to disguise the identities of the individuals involved. Nevertheless, the authors,
editors and publishers can make no warranties that the information contained herein
is totally free from error, not least because clinical standards are constantly changing
through research and regulation. The authors, editors and publishers therefore
disclaim all liability for direct or consequential damages resulting from the use of
material contained in this book. Readers are strongly advised to pay careful attention
to information provided by the manufacturer of any drugs or equipment that they plan
to use.

Contents

Preface

Becoming smoke free is a radical lifestyle change. Assisting smokers in successfully making that change is a highly rewarding endeavor for health professionals providing smoking cessation interventions. It is rewarding to witness the transformation clients go through as they gradually extract themselves from the stranglehold nicotine has on their daily routines and embrace the fresh outlook on their lives that lies ahead on the smoke-free path. It is also gratifying to know that for each smoker who is helped to stay smoke free, there are others in that person's life who are happy and relieved to see their loved one choose health over debilitating habit. Of course, the benefits of becoming smoke free go beyond the individuals seeking treatment. Smoking cessation providers play a key role in improving public health.

The social and political context in which smoking occurs has dramatically changed over the last few decades. The numbers of daily smokers have been steadily declining in many countries (e.g., daily smoking rates for Australians aged 14 years and older have declined by 40% between 1985 and 2004 alone, with now fewer than one in five persons smoking daily [Australian Institute of Health and Welfare, 2007]). In parallel with this trend, an increasing number of nations have enacted legislation prohibiting smoking in public buildings, restaurants, pubs, and many workplaces, and restricting it to special areas segregated from the smoke-free mainstream. Importantly, smoking has become socially stigmatized, and tolerance for suffering exposure to second-hand smoke has been replaced by firm policies to protect the non-smoking public from smoking-related health risks. It is in this changed environment of stigmatization and social pressures that many smokers who have difficulty quitting on their own seek the help of trained professionals. To meet that demand, health professionals must combine compassion for the plight of these "hard-core" smokers with rigor in the application of science-informed intervention strategies.

It is little more than a decade ago that empirically supported treatment approaches for nicotine dependence became broadly available via the systematic dissemination of clinical practice guidelines. For the busy healthcare professional, it is, however, a big step from adopting practice *guidelines* to knowing how to put these guidelines into *practice*. The task is further complicated when a group of clients is the intervention target rather than an individual client. This manual was developed to help service providers with less experience in running groups to conduct an effective group intervention for smoking cessation. The manual has two aims: (a) to translate international clinical practice guidelines into step-by-step instructions for setting up, conducting, and evaluating a group intervention for smoking cessation; and (b) to provide ready-to-use client materials and treatment tools. The core content areas and treatment strategies covered in the manual are consistent with the *Standard for Training in Smoking Cessation Treatments* for group interventions published by the Health Development Agency in the UK in 2003.

We would like to thank Bruce Campbell for sharing his dual expertise as a pharmacist and clinical psychologist on pharmacological aids to smoking cessation. We also would like to acknowledge a few colleagues whose feedback was instrumental in the development and refinement of some of the materials in this manual: Casey Ashby, Emma-Jane Barclay, Beatrice Drysdale, Nichola Forster, Rebecca Jamieson, Kristy Johnstone, Fiona Michel, Claire Nulsen, Georgie Paulik, Rikki Prott, Michael Stephens, and Leanne Wheat.

Introduction and overview of program

Smoking is a leading cause of preventable disease and deaths in developed countries such as Australia, the USA, and the UK. Like other addictions, it has proved difficult to treat and is associated with high relapse rates. Abstinence rates have been reported to be as low as 22% six months after treatment (Fiore *et al.*, 1994) and are even lower after unaided quit attempts (Garvey *et al.*, 1992). Although there is no shortage of self-help materials designed to reach a large proportion of smokers, available evidence suggests that self-administered treatments are only effective when combined with supportive interventions (Curry, Ludman, & McClure, 2003). In recent years, significant progress has been made in the development and dissemination of clinical practice guidelines on the basis of systematic reviews of empirically supported treatment approaches (Fiore *et al.*, 2000; Miller & Wood, 2002; Raw, McNeill, & West, 1998; West, McNeill, & Raw, 2000). In addition, many governments and health authorities maintain web-based resources for health professionals that inform about current developments in evidence-based smoking cessation services and products (e.g., an excellent website is maintained by the Smoking Cessation Service Research Network in the UK; www.scsrn.org). There are also some treatment handbooks and manuals available (e.g., Abrams *et al.*, 2003; McEwen *et al.*, 2006) that convey essential background information on smoking-related issues and offer practical guidance for those involved in smoking cessation. These manuals, however, focus primarily on providing cessation services to individuals and typically devote only a single chapter to group interventions.

Group-based formats have success rates that are comparable to individual treatments, but they have the advantage that they reach more people. Hence, group programs are particularly well suited for the cost-effective delivery of intense multicomponent treatments that guide smokers through the phases of preparing for change, quitting, and maintaining a smoke-free lifestyle. However, group interventions present broader conceptual and practical challenges to health professionals who deliver them than interventions that are tailored to only one client. This *Treatment Manual for Smoking Cessation Groups* describes how to meet these challenges successfully. It provides detailed guidance on how to run an evidence-based smoking cessation program in a group format.

This manual has been designed with the busy professional in mind. It is meant for use by healthcare professionals who want to offer group-based smoking cessation programs but may be limited in their time and resources to translate and adapt recommendations from best practice guidelines and comprehensive treatment handbooks into a succinct manual that is ready to use, incorporates up-to-date practice guidelines, and can be administered to clients with a great degree of flexibility. The flexible administration allows the treatment to be tailored towards the concerns and needs of the current group members on a session-by-session basis. Because smoking cessation programs tend to be offered in a variety of settings by a broad spectrum of health professionals with diverse training backgrounds, each of the modules in the program provides the therapist with brief background information and easy to follow guidelines regarding the treatment aims and principles relevant to that module. The *Therapist guidelines* section of each module is followed by a complementary section with *Client materials*, containing handouts and worksheets to be used with the clients. These materials facilitate the introduction of program elements and strategies in a client-focused, easy-to-understand format during sessions, and also serve as "self-help" materials for initiating, monitoring, and sustaining clients' change processes between sessions. The program elements and strategies reflect the core elements of intense multicomponent smoking cessation interventions recommended by international best practice guidelines, as well as by general principles underlying evidence-based treatments for addictive behaviors (e.g., Miller & Heather, 1998).

Core elements of the multicomponent smoking cessation program

Combining behavioral and pharmacological approaches

Nicotine addiction is not only maintained by the reinforcing pharmacological effects of the drug, but it is also powerfully reinforced by the behavioral aspects of the addiction. Consequently, both the pharmacological and behavioral components of this addiction need to be addressed in treatment. The behavioral addiction is so powerful because smoking incidents typically occur very frequently over the course of a day. Each incident involves a number of puffs – each of which can be thought of as a learning trial (O'Brien, 1997). For a regular smoker, this results in thousands of learning trials every month that strongly link smoking with many everyday activities such as eating, drinking, and driving. Cues associated with these links can produce and maintain a strong desire to smoke (Droungas et al., 1995). To break the behavioral addiction, these associations between everyday cues and smoking must be disrupted. At the same time, new associations need to be learned that link these everyday cues with smoke-free activities. Therefore, from day one of the program, clients are encouraged to engage in a process of "re-wiring" the connections between routine behaviors and smoke-free cues.

The pharmacological component of the addiction has an equally strong grip on the smoker's life. This is because the pharmacological actions of nicotine produce their reinforcing effects in the brain within seconds of smoking a cigarette (Benowitz, 1996). Tolerance to these desired effects tends to develop quickly, and hence more cigarettes are needed to achieve the same effects. Moreover, following cessation of smoking, many smokers experience unpleasant nicotine withdrawal symptoms (Hughes, 2007; Shiffman et al., 2006). To break the chemical addiction, pharmacotherapy can assist in gradually weaning off the clients from the chemical rewards associated with nicotine, while attenuating the impact of any withdrawal distress. The evidence shows that pharmacological treatments approximately double quitting rates when compared with a placebo, and that there can be added benefits of combining pharmacotherapy with behavioral interventions (Mooney & Hatsukami, 2001).

Setting a low threshold for initiating the process of behavior change

One of the benefits of combining pharmacological and behavioral approaches stems from the ability to select from a range of evidence-based strategies. This provides a menu of options allowing clients to engage first in those strategies they find most appealing and easiest to maintain. Hence, the threshold for taking the first steps on the arduous journey of becoming smoke free is deliberately set low. The most important aim at this stage is to get the change process going. Once under way, promoting clients' self-efficacy regarding their ability to make progressive changes to their smoking behaviors becomes an integral part of the process. The emphasis throughout the treatment program is on becoming smoke free for good, rather than on quitting as the immediate goal.

Part of this process is to develop an understanding of the quitting process. The initial focus is on weakening the strength of the behavioral addiction. This is based on the simple rationale that behavior change occurs from doing things differently. Of the many everyday things that a client can start doing differently to disrupt the established behavior–smoking associations, the one or two that present as the least challenging are targeted first. Given the relatively low difficulty of achieving these targets, the likelihood of experiencing success is high. This will, in turn, boost the clients' motivation and confidence for tackling the more difficult step of quitting smoking altogether. Because these behavioral changes disrupt typical smoking routines, some reduction – however small – in the amount of cigarettes smoked per day is almost inevitable. It is empowering for clients to become aware of how these subtle changes in the amount and pattern of their smoking are the result of their own efforts at doing things differently. Therefore, a simple behavioral monitoring exercise is introduced from day one of the treatment program. This method enables smokers to begin to develop some sense of control over their addiction before quitting. An added benefit for those smokers who reduce their cigarette use during this period by more than 50% is that it increases their chances of becoming smoke free (Hughes, 2000). Once the threshold for continued efforts to engage in behaviors that are uncoupled from smoking has been crossed, clients are encouraged to set a quit date for a time when they will feel ready. At this time, they will also be coached in pharmacological treatment options. With this dual approach, the need for the chemical nicotine fix can then be gradually weakened, while new behaviors associated with a smoke-free lifestyle become more and more established.

Personalizing treatment: providing a menu of options

Most smokers quit on their own without the support of formal intervention programs. Not every former smoker has used the same strategy for becoming smoke free. Likewise, within the range of evidence-based strategies recommended by clinical practice guidelines, there is much scope for flexibility and choice. For example, there now exists a variety of effective nicotine-replacement therapies such as nicotine patches, gum, nasal spray, inhalers, and lozenges. What type to chose may be influenced by contraindications such as pregnancy, breastfeeding, or allergies, but for the most part can be left to smoker preferences (Goldstein, 2003). Similarly, among the behavioral strategies available for disrupting the automaticity of daily smoking routines, there is an even greater selection to choose from. The key here is to match each client with a personalized set of behavior change tools that will work for the client. After all, it is the client who must wield the tools and do the changing.

The principle of providing a menu of options has a firm basis in the general literature on motivational interventions for substance misuse (Bien, Miller, & Tonigan, 1993). One critical element common to effective motivational interventions is an emphasis on communicating that change is the client's responsibility and choice (Miller, 1995). For smokers to embrace that responsibility and perceive that they have a choice, it is essential to offer them a menu of alternative strategies from which to choose. The chances of becoming smoke free on a particular attempt without the aid of formal treatments are no higher than about 3% (Jarvis & Sutherland, 1998). This low success rate attests to the difficulty of the struggle faced by smokers who wish to become smoke free. A menu of options increases the likelihood that every smoker will find some strategies that they are comfortable with and ready to give a try. This also provides hope in the face of previous failures to quit, which, in turn, can provide an energizing boost to the motivation to become smoke free.

Enhancing motivation to become smoke free

There are many reasons why people want to kick their smoking habit. Some want to change because they value the benefits that a smoke-free life can bring. Others are prompted by external factors. They may be jolted into action by the worried pleas of their children and loved ones, a stern warning by a doctor, an alarming prognosis after a recent medical check-up, a close brush with death following a smoking-related emergency hospitalization, or the guilt stemming from exposing others to the hazards of environmental tobacco smoke. In recent years, external pressures to quit have even further intensified, as bans on smoking in public places are becoming the norm, and being a smoker carries an increasingly negative stigma. But ultimately, none of these "good" reasons will lead someone to become smoke free unless that person believes that these reasons outweigh the perceived benefits of smoking, as well as make up for the perceived negative consequences of quitting. Reaching that decision point, making a commitment to change, and sustaining that commitment through the tribulations of lapses and relapses require smokers to be highly motivated. Moreover, the motives that lead smokers to initiate change may be different from the motives that help them to maintain that change (Rothman, 2000). Therefore, monitoring and enhancing motivation to become smoke free is an integral part of this treatment program.

Accounting for progress and rewarding every successful step

Once smokers have crossed the threshold for initiating change and have begun to tackle some behavioral strategies from a menu of options, it is critical that these efforts and their effects are accurately monitored, and that clients receive continuous feedback on their progress. This is important for two reasons. First, involving clients in self-monitoring helps them to become aware of specific aspects of their routine behaviors that challenge current assumptions about their behavior. This information is instrumental in promoting self-evaluation and decision making in the change process (DiClemente, 2003). Second, because the ultimate goal of long-term abstinence is a dichotomous outcome, this poses too high a hurdle to serve as a sensitive measure to evaluate treatment success (Hughes, 2002). If treatment success is solely evaluated against the gold standard of long-term abstinence, clients may experience any delays in progressing toward that goal as failure. In contrast, accounting for progress on intermediate measures (e.g., fewer numbers of cigarettes smoked each week) allows clients to experience success. This will be instrumental in enhancing motivation to persist with efforts to reach the more difficult and distal goal of maintaining a smoke-free lifestyle. Moreover, there is evidence that a reduction in the number of cigarettes smoked per day can improve health if it is not accompanied by increases in the intensity of smoking of the remaining cigarettes (Godtfredsen *et al.*, 2002). The impact of compensatory smoking on net health benefits achieved by cigarette fading can be assessed by monitoring changes in a biomarker of toxin exposure such as carbon monoxide. Receiving feedback on reductions in average carbon monoxide level is a tangible indicator of progress and can be a powerful motivator for clients along the way to long-term abstinence.

For clients to benefit fully from the gradual changes that occur because of their successful implementation of behavior change strategies, they must be aware of these changes. Some of these changes will be subtle at first and become obvious only when viewed as a trend over repeated measurements. Hence, progress is best communicated to the client by illustrating their successful steps in the change process through graphing (Page & Stritzke, 2006; Woody *et al.*, 2003). Visual representations of whether the things that a client attempts to "do differently" result in a change in smoking behavior, or whether things stay the same, will be illuminating for the individual. Thus, inspection of progress with the help of clear graphs is a routine component of each session in this treatment program. It also provides opportunities for vicarious learning by observing the progress patterns of other group members, and the graphical feedback feels like a reward for the time spent recording the data (Woody *et al.*, 2003).

Delivering treatment at a high level of intensity

There is a strong dose–response relation between intensity of treatment delivery and cessation success (Fiore *et al.*, 2000). Greater cessation rates are achieved with longer session length and a higher number of sessions. Treatments lasting more than eight sessions have the highest abstinence rates. Only a minority of smokers achieve permanent abstinence in an initial quit attempt, and most will experience a relapse within two weeks after quitting (Garvey *et al.*, 1992). Therefore, the treatment program consists of 10 weekly sessions to allow for a period of continued support following individual quit dates, which are typically set around half-way through the program. In addition, because tobacco dependence shows many features of a chronic disease, a follow-up session is recommended (Fiore *et al.*, 2000). This will provide an opportunity to congratulate sustained success or, if tobacco use has occurred, to review circumstances and encourage recommitment to the goal of becoming smoke free.

Promoting lifestyle change

Quitting is one thing, becoming smoke free is quite another, and remaining smoke free involves a fairly dramatic lifestyle change. Promoting lifestyle change as a successful aid to remaining smoke free is an important focus of the program. This aspect of the program acknowledges the grief process and far-reaching changes that often occur in a person's life as a result of giving up smoking. The language used within the modules of this manual and in conducting the treatment program is carefully chosen to help smokers to see the changes they are making as something positive rather than negative. That is, instead of describing the change they are undertaking as "quitting" smoking, with its negative connotations of losing something, it is instead described as "becoming smoke free." Becoming smoke free signals a process of gaining something. Participants are gaining the freedom to make lifestyle choices unfettered by the demands of nicotine dependence.

Incorporating the idea of lifestyle change in this program also acknowledges that smoking has played a significant role in the life of a smoker and that new activities, beliefs, and coping strategies are going to be needed to take the place of the "smoking lifestyle." The module on lifestyle change helps participants to reduce the risk of relapse through, first, developing an awareness of how imbalances in lifestyle and some aspects of a person's previous lifestyle choices (before becoming smoke free) can threaten their attempts to remain abstinent (Marlatt & Gordon, 1985), and, second, adopting ways to address these imbalances in order to promote a smoke-free lifestyle.

Integrating individual treatment planning with facilitation of group processes

Treatment planning is an essential element of accountable practice. In group-based interventions, treatment planning involves two aspects. One is the individual case conceptualization that follows from the synthesis and integration of the assessment information regarding each individual smoker's history and circumstances. The other aspect is a "group conceptualization." That is, treatment planning takes into account the unique constellation of characteristics and circumstances for individual group members. The aim is to anticipate and plan for likely patterns of group interactions and processes that can either hinder or facilitate individual client's treatment goals. The group format has the additional benefit of securing social support as part of treatment.

Treatments for smoking cessation that incorporate supportive interventions are associated with superior outcomes (Fiore *et al.*, 2000). Hence, the purposive integration of individual treatment plans with the supportive elements arising from the dynamics within a particular group is an important task throughout the program.

Communicating caring and empathy

With the implementation of smoking bans in public places such as restaurants, airports, and workplaces, smoking has become an increasingly stigmatized behavior. Health promotion campaigns often use in-your-face strategies to portray smokers as unattractive, not smart, uncool, and plagued by bad smell and poor health. The image of sophistication, sex appeal, fun, and adventure traditionally associated with smoking has been largely replaced by connotations of disgust or pity. Many smokers joining a smoking cessation program report of their feelings of frustration and shame stemming from other people's negative reactions to their smoking habit. These can run the gamut from openly expressed hostility to more subtle reactions perceived as resentment, rejection, or disappointment. It is against the backdrop of this climate of disapproval that smokers encounter the staff conducting the smoking cessation program. From the outset, it will be very important that treatment staff are sensitive to these issues and foster supportive and caring interactions (Fiore *et al.*, 2000). There is strong evidence that skillful communication of empathic understanding improves success rates in treatment for addictive behaviors (Miller, 1998). The emphasis is on a collaborative approach, where the smoker is encouraged to be a full partner in the development of the treatment plan (Abrams & Niaura, 2003). The role of the therapist in this collaboration is similar to a "coach" (Greenberg, 2002), using language that is valuing and appreciative to help clients to progress toward their goal of becoming smoke free. There is evidence that such a collaborative "group-oriented" approach, rather than a more didactic "therapist-oriented" approach, facilitates better long-term outcomes for smokers (Hajek, Belcher, & Stapleton, 1985). Consequently, it is important that the language therapists use conveys this collaborative, caring, and empathic approach.

Incorporating humor

Smoking is a serious health risk. Overcoming the dual stranglehold of instant chemical gratification and strong behavioral habit requires a serious commitment. Hence, becoming smoke free poses a serious challenge, and failing to meet this challenge successfully can have serious consequences. Despite the anxiety, guilt, shame, and high stakes that prompt smokers to seek help from a smoking cessation program, the journey of becoming smoke free must not be drudgery. Therapists are encouraged to incorporate a healthy dose of humor throughout the treatment program. This can go a long way in helping clients to cope with this difficult lifestyle transition and maintain a positive outlook in the face of temporary setbacks.

Overview of the program

The program is designed to run for 10 weekly sessions, each of two hours' duration, plus a follow-up session one month after treatment. Prior to the group commencing, an individual assessment session for each group member is scheduled (Figure 1.1).

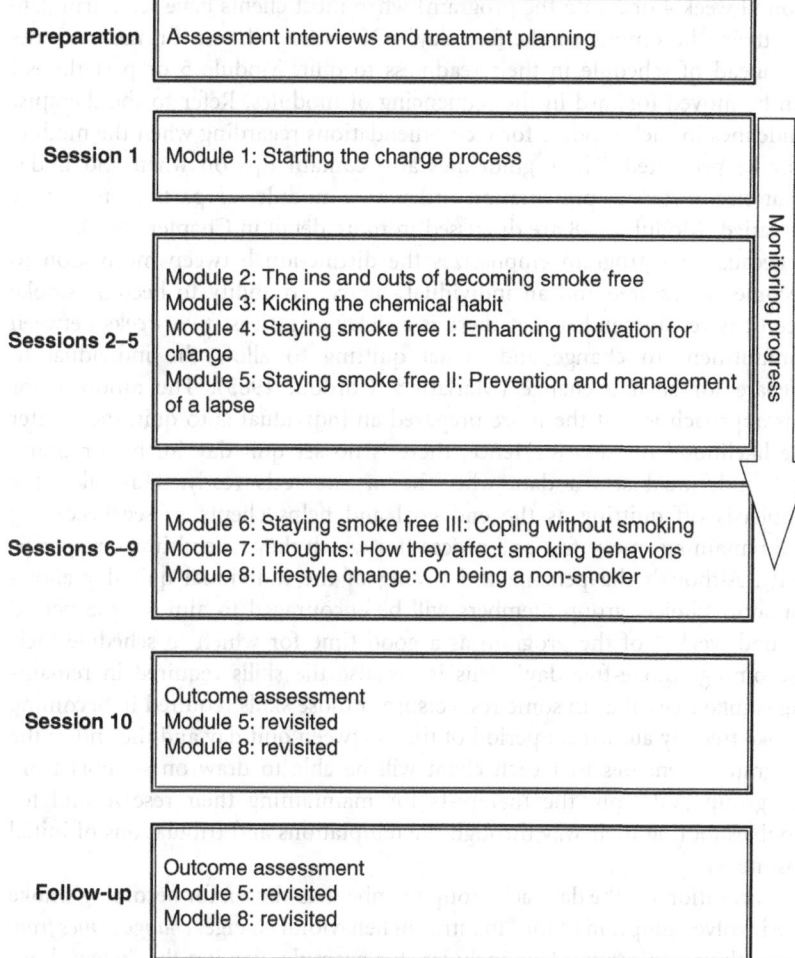

| **Preparation** | Assessment interviews and treatment planning |

| **Session 1** | Module 1: Starting the change process |

| **Sessions 2–5** | Module 2: The ins and outs of becoming smoke free
Module 3: Kicking the chemical habit
Module 4: Staying smoke free I: Enhancing motivation for change
Module 5: Staying smoke free II: Prevention and management of a lapse |

| **Sessions 6–9** | Module 6: Staying smoke free III: Coping without smoking
Module 7: Thoughts: How they affect smoking behaviors
Module 8: Lifestyle change: On being a non-smoker |

| **Session 10** | Outcome assessment
Module 5: revisited
Module 8: revisited |

| **Follow-up** | Outcome assessment
Module 5: revisited
Module 8: revisited |

Monitoring progress

Figure 1.1 Overview of program and approximate timing of modules.

The manual is structured in a flexible manner that enables the therapists to determine which module is most appropriate to cover each week. The exception to this is that the first session should cover the module *Starting the change process*. This module provides an outline of the rationale on which the program is based and is designed to engage group members in active change from the outset. It is also recommended that the following modules be covered in the earlier sessions: *The ins and outs of becoming smoke free, Kicking the chemical habit*, and *Staying smoke free I: enhancing the motivation*. Note that some sections in later modules build on progress achieved in previous sessions. For example, the section *What to do when a lapse occurs* in Module 5 becomes most relevant around the time (usually around week 4 or 5 into the program) when most clients have set a firm date for their "becoming smoke-free day." Of course, if one or more clients are ahead of schedule in their readiness to quit, Module 5 or part thereof can be moved forward in the sequencing of modules. Refer to the therapist guidelines in each module for recommendations regarding when the module may be presented. These guidelines also contain tips on when and under what circumstances presentation order of a module, or parts thereof, may be varied. Modules 1–8 are discussed in more detail in Chapters 3–10.

Because the program emphasizes the distinction between motivation to become smoke free and an individual's perceived ability to become smoke free, it is recommended that there is a delay of at least two weeks between commitment to change and actual quitting to allow the individual to prepare for such a change (Marlatt & Gordon, 1985). The rationale for this approach is that the more prepared an individual is to quit, the greater the likelihood of success. Hence, there is no set quit day in this program: each individual sets a date when he or she feels ready. This takes the emphasis off quitting as the end goal and helps clients to see becoming and remaining smoke free as a process for which they take ultimate responsibility. Although the personalized timing of the individual quit day allows for some choice, group members will be encouraged to aim for the period around week 4 of the program as a good time for which to schedule their "becoming smoke-free day." This is because the skills required in remaining smoke free differ in some respects from those skills required in becoming smoke free. By allowing a period of time between quit day and the end of the program, it ensures that each client will be able to draw on support from the group and from the therapists for maintaining their resolve and for troubleshooting their way through the temptations and tribulations of initial abstinence.

Preparation for the day each group member has chosen for becoming smoke free involves adoption of the "mantra" of behavioral change: *change comes from doing things differently*. This includes, for example, varying the "when, how, where" for each smoking behavior. Group members are coached to use these behavioral strategies to decrease the amount of cigarettes smoked continually. A checklist for some of these strategies is included in the *Starting the change process* module. It is strongly recommended that these be introduced in the first session and revisited weekly throughout the program. Group members should endeavor to adopt at least two strategies each week, and to keep a tally of the number of days that these strategies were used and the number of cigarettes they smoked during each day. This process of self-monitoring is an important aspect of the change process. It allows group members to observe changes over time, and the process of monitoring often itself leads to behavioral changes. Another benefit of self-monitoring is that it allows the therapists and the group to reinforce *any* changes – however small – in the right direction.

The end of the program should be marked with recognition of the group members' progress along the journey to be smoke free. It is suggested that a certificate be awarded to each member indicating that they have come to possess skills that will help them on their journey as a non-smoker (see the final module: *Lifestyle change: on being a non-smoker*).

Structure of sessions

The first half of each session should begin with a discussion of the self-monitoring of strategies and events related to smoking over the previous week. The second half of the session should then focus on one of the skill-acquisition modules. The idea is to select the module (or parts of modules) that best addresses those issues emerging from the personalized discussion during the first half of the sessions. There may be occasions when it is best to revisit parts of modules already covered before introducing new modules, depending on the pattern of individual and group progress. Finally, try to end each session with an imagery exercise to facilitate group members' ability to develop a new self-image as a non-smoker. There are a few such exercises included in the manual and others can be developed based on the preferences of group members (i.e., what personal changes and benefits they envisage as a result of being smoke free). It is recommended to end the first session with the imagery exercise contrasting life before and after smoking (*Smoke City versus Fresh Hills*).

Tips for working with individuals

Although this manual is specifically designed for delivering a smoking cessation program in a group format, the program can also be used one on one when working with individuals. The client materials are client centered, but where they do make references to a group context, clients in individual treatment can be instructed to ignore those. With respect to the therapist guidelines, they will be simplified as there is no need to accommodate simultaneously the diverse characteristics and change trajectories of multiple group members. To help users of this manual to make the relevant adjustments when applying it in a one-on-one treatment context, each chapter has at the end of the guidelines a textbox of tips for working with individuals. These textboxes highlight how certain elements of the treatment modules can be adapted from the group format so they are readily applicable to a single client.

Assessment, treatment planning, and evaluation of outcomes

THERAPIST GUIDELINES

Aims

1 Gather information about each client's smoking history and other core dimensions relevant to making the change from being a smoker to leading a life that is smoke free
2 Identify client characteristics and circumstances that may either facilitate or potentially hinder group processes
3 Arrive at a treatment plan by (a) conceptualizing which individual client characteristics are optimally addressed by which components of the treatment program, and (b) anticipating how the client's individual features could be best brought into play in maximizing the benefit of group processes
4 Establish rapport and a spirit of collaboration
5 Establish a baseline against which progress and outcomes can be evaluated.

Assessment for a smoking cessation group has two primary functions: (a) collecting an individual case history, and (b) preparing the individual client for the group. Both of these aims can be achieved with a structured interview. The template for the interview is reproduced in the second part of this chapter, which contains the *Therapist materials*. In the following sections, we guide you through the different parts of the interview, and how to use the information for the purpose of individual case formulation and group preparation.

Problem identification and case formulation

Introduction and referral information

After the brief introduction, which orients the client to the aims of the interview, the first step is to gather the referral information. Reasons and circumstances for seeking treatment can vary considerably across clients. This variability has implications for the motivation clients bring to the task of becoming smoke free and their likelihood of successfully engaging in the treatment. For example, clients who like smoking but feel pressured to quit smoking by an employer who is concerned about the corporate image are often less committed to change than clients who want to quit smoking because they are disgusted by their habit and are concerned about their own health. That is, if the motivation for change comes from *within* the person, there is a greater likelihood that the person will sustain the motivation to change and stay smoke free. In contrast, if the motivation for change comes from *outside* the person, readiness for change can easily be undermined by a personally held desire to continue smoking.

The second question about *what the client wants to achieve* by coming to this group is designed to elicit more detail following the more general question of *what brings you here*, but more importantly, it focuses the client from the very start on *outcomes*! It communicates clearly to the client that this group is about achieving specific outcomes, and that the client has the responsibility of setting a realistic target for himself or herself.

Although there is a great deal of variability in the reasons people give to quit smoking, there will also be similarities across members of the group. Identifying these similarities is helpful in structuring the first and subsequent treatment sessions, because one can use common themes to facilitate inter-actions between group members and initiate peer support. For example, if three group members have medical problems associated with smoking and have been told by their doctors that continuing to smoke will complicate recovery, hasten rapid decline in health, or, worse, increase the imminent risk of premature death, these clients can be encouraged to share their experiences and support each other in achieving a change toward a healthier lifestyle. Other clients may share a concern about setting a bad example to their young children, exposing them to secondary smoke, or causing them distress through their belief that their parent may die a premature death. Motive clusters like these can be used skillfully by the group therapists to generate quick rapport and cohesion among group members in the first two sessions of the program.

Pattern and context of cigarette smoking

The first two questions ask about the *onset of smoking*. This provides insight into how chronic the problem is. Identification of the circumstances at onset also can offer clues about what secondary function smoking may have served in the past. For example, to "fit in" with work colleagues, to "cope" with a stressful life event, or to "feel glamorous" when hitting the night clubs, are all perceived gains associated with smoking. If eliminated by smoking cessation, the clients need to learn during treatment how these aspects can be achieved in alternative ways without smoking. For older clients, reflecting for a moment about the circumstances of their onset of smoking often sharpens the realization of how things have changed in relation to smoking, and how their habit has caused them to be "out of step" with contemporary attitudes and lifestyle practices. This can provide an additional motivational boost for getting serious about becoming smoke free.

The next two items *quantify the extent of nicotine use*. Number of cigarettes and money spent are different quantitative indicators of the severity of smoking. Both indices can be easily monitored by clients during treatment on a daily basis. Hence, these measures provide a powerful tool for demonstrating even small (and rewarding!) changes in nicotine use as clients begin to put cessation strategies into practice.

The question about *pack size* serves two functions. First, it draws the focus on actual numbers of cigarettes contained in a pack. Many clients use this as a "benchmark" to keep track of their cigarette use in a given day. Second, it will reveal if clients buy cigarettes in bulk to save money. Changing buying habits to disrupt smoking-related routines and to reduce availability of cigarettes to "one pack at a time" is one of the behavioral treatment targets early in the group program.

The question about the *nicotine level* often reveals if clients believe the myth that lower-strength cigarettes are less harmful to their health, which can be used as an early opportunity to educate them about the pitfalls of compensatory smoking (Box 2.1).

Box 2.1. Compensatory smoking

- Compensatory smoking can occur when smokers attempt to reduce their nicotine intake by reducing the number of cigarettes they smoke per day or by switching to so-called "mild", low-yield brands.
- Because smokers are used to a regular amount of nicotine, they subconsciously adjust their smoking behavior so that they can still receive similar amounts of nicotine.
- Smokers can compensate for the lower nicotine intake by smoking the fewer (or "milder") cigarettes more intensely. They do this by (a) taking longer puffs, (b) taking more puffs, (c) smoking to a shorter butt length, and (d) inhaling the smoke for longer.[1]
- Smokers can also compensate for the filter ventilation used in lower tar cigarettes by behaviorally blocking the vents with their fingers or lips.[1,2]
- Compensation is typically partial.[3] That is, some net reduction in overall exposure to nicotine, carbon monoxide, and tobacco carcinogens occurs with smoking fewer or "lighter" cigarettes, but unless this reduction exceeds 50%, health risks are not appreciably reduced.[4] Smoking lower

Box 2.1 (cont.)

tar cigarettes is not safer or healthier than smoking regular cigarettes. This is a myth created by industry advertising.[5]

- Some newer cigarettes use genetically modified tobacco to provide a nicotine step-down approach by varying the nicotine content from high to very low while delivering equivalent levels of tar. Because of compensatory smoking, CO exposure is higher in the low nicotine product than the high nicotine product. Consequently, although these genetically modified cigarettes are marketed as "potential reduced exposure products (PREPS)," evidence suggest that they instead may be a harm-increasing product.[6]
- The level of compensatory smoking can be addressed in treatment with the use of a biomarker such as CO by establishing a baseline of CO exposure at the assessment interview and then monitoring CO levels throughout the treatment program and at follow-up. If significant reductions in smoking are not accompanied by proportional reductions in CO exposure, this may be a result of compensatory smoking behaviors. Raising awareness of these behaviors can help clients to minimize them, and it also serves as a reminder that reduction in smoking is only a step on the way to becoming smoke free, with only the latter achieving maximum health benefits.

Sources: 1. Kozlowski & O'Connor, 2002; 2. Rose & Behm, 2004; 3. Scherer, 1999; 4. Bollinger *et al.*, 2002; 5. King *et al.*, 2003; 6. Strasser *et al.*, 2007.

The next question, *"How soon after you wake up do you smoke your first cigarette?"* is an efficient and reliable way to measure nicotine dependence (Heatherton *et al.*, 1991). Time to first cigarette of the day is the strongest behavioral predictor of nicotine dependence. It correlates closely with nicotine levels as measured by the biomarker cotinine, a nicotinic metabolite most commonly measured in saliva (Jarvis & Sutherland, 1998), and it is the best self-report index of genetic vulnerability to nicotine dependence (Haberstick *et al.*, 2007). Smokers who light up within 30 minutes of waking are considered more dependent than smokers who take longer until smoking their first cigarette. For these "early morning smokers," more intense cognitive–behavioral interventions and higher-dose pharmacological treatments are beneficial (Niaura & Shadel, 2003). They are also most likely to experience a range of withdrawal symptoms. The question about the time to the first cigarette of the day is taken from the six-item Fagerström Test for Nicotine Dependence (FTND, Heatherton *et al.*, 1991). It is often desirable to administer the full version of the FTND for diagnostic and outcome monitoring purposes. The FTND is brief and easy to score and is included in the *Therapist materials.* Scores can range from 0 to 10, with higher scores indicating higher levels of dependence. A score of 6 or greater is usually considered a high level of dependence.

The next question asks about what (if any) *withdrawal symptoms* the client has experienced in the past. Although many smokers report withdrawal symptoms following the cessation of smoking, not everyone does, and for some they are only mildly distressing. Symptoms include irritability, frustration, anger, restlessness, difficulty concentrating, light-headedness, disturbed sleep, anxiety, depressed mood, cravings for cigarettes, and increased appetite. It is important to reassure clients that these symptoms peak in intensity within the first week after smoking the last cigarette, and most will disappear over three or four weeks (Hughes, 2007; Shiffman *et al.*, 2006). Only urges to smoke and increased appetite may last for several months after becoming smoke free. Using nicotine-replacement strategies can alleviate the severity of withdrawal. Therefore, clients who report high levels of withdrawal distress are especially good candidates for using nicotine replacement to reduce the risk of relapse during the month following cessation.

The remaining set of questions in this section collects *information about recent and past smoke-free periods.* Details are recorded about (a) longest time without a cigarette in the last week and year, (b) previous use (if any) of nicotine-replacement treatments or bupropion (Zyban), (c) recency and duration of last quit attempt, (d) strategies previously found helpful by the client, and (e) duration of current level of smoking. These details about the nature and variability of previous quit attempts and smoke-free periods can be very useful in treatment planning. For example, learning that a female client was able to quit "cold-turkey" and stay smoke free for nine months during pregnancy, or that a client remained smoke free for two years during an extended overseas stay with a non-smoking companion, or that another client has never been smoke free for more than an hour for the past 20 years except when on airplanes, makes for a diverse mix of client experiences with being smoke free. Change is always easier when one can draw on previous experiences with having changed successfully in the past than when one enters completely unfamiliar territory. Likewise, strategies that proved unsuccessful in the past, such as going "cold turkey" without also using nicotine replacement, or the experience of side effects when taking medication such as bupropion, can be avoided. Thus, information about previous successes and failures can be helpful when working out what treatment strategies are best suited for which client(s) in the group.

Motivation for change and potential barriers to change

Becoming smoke free is a difficult task. Clients typically consider joining a group for smoking cessation because attempts on their own, even with the help of pharmacological treatments, have repeatedly failed in the past. For them to decide "to give it a go" is an important step, but it does not necessarily mean their motivation for change and their confidence that they will stay the course is consistently strong. In light of perceived barriers to change, motivation to engage in treatment is highly variable across and within clients. Indeed, some clients will change their mind about their readiness after the assessment interview and not show up for the first group session. Without motivation to work hard to succeed, any strategies on offer for helping to become smoke free will be undermined or ineffectual. It is, therefore, essential to assess and monitor client's motivation for initiating and maintaining change throughout. This information will direct treatment planning to ensure that motivational strength and commitment are targeted for intervention whenever a client show signs of waning commitment or frustration with setbacks.

The first question in this section asks the client *"how likely do you think it is that you will be a non-smoker in six months' time?"* This is a simple way of gauging the client's confidence in reaching the stated goal. The follow-up question to probe for reasons why the client gave his or her particular rating is often helpful in gaining insight into what the client perceives as potential barriers or facilitating circumstances that either undermine or boost the chance of success.

The next question assesses *readiness for change*. This provides an indication of how committed the client is to work hard to make the switch from being a smoker to being a non-smoker. In addition, from a group perspective, clients who report low readiness for change can have a negative and demoralizing impact on group interactions. Therefore, prior knowledge of who shows low readiness for change is helpful in monitoring and preempting any negative impact they may have on other group members.

The next two questions identify *occasions where it is particularly difficult or relatively easy to abstain from smoking*. This information guides individualized treatment planning in terms of which cigarettes during the daily smoking routine a client might tackle first when beginning to cut down on their cigarette use, leaving the more difficult occasions for later. It may also provide valuable information about high-risk situations and environmental cues that the client can learn to avoid or cope with. For example, some modules in the treatment program are designed to help clients to strengthen their refusal skills and assertiveness.

The next two questions identify sources of environmental barriers and social support for becoming smoke free. Living with someone who smokes is a strong predictor of poor treatment outcome, whereas the likelihood of success can be enhanced by a supportive network of family, friends, and colleagues (Chandola, Head, & Bartley, 2004; Walsh *et al.*, 2007).

The final two questions in this section assess the *level of ambivalence toward change*. Motivation for change is not all or none. It is common among clients in smoking cessation programs to experience some ambivalence toward making such a profound lifestyle change. It would be naive to expect that, the desire to still smoke suddenly vanishes into thin air when people develop the desire to *not* smoke, which is a strong motivating force for joining a smoking cessation group. Ambivalence, or feeling two ways about something, is a good intermediate state to be in for someone who is attempting to move from a chronic, non-ambivalent behavioral pattern (i.e., "pure approach" evident in heavy smoking behavior unchecked by any serious inclinations to avoid smoking) all the way to a permanent, smoke-free behavioral pattern (i.e., "pure avoidance" as evident in complete abstinence from smoking untroubled by any residual inclinations to return to smoking). In motivational interviewing terms (Miller, 1998), the process of moving a client from a pure approach motivation to a consolidated avoidance motivation via motivational ambivalence is referred to as "developing a discrepancy." That is, clients are helped to see an incompatibility between their current behavior and choices (i.e., smoking) and a desired goal (e.g., reducing risk of dying from a diagnosed lung condition). As the relative balance shifts from approach to avoidance, the likelihood of treatment success increases. Conversely, to the extent that the strength of approach inclinations outweighs the strength of avoidance inclinations, the likelihood of failure to stop smoking or relapse is high (Stritzke *et al.*, 2004; cf. Stritzke *et al.*, 2007).

To obtain a quantitative measure of the client's ambivalence toward change, first explain the simple metaphor of "two voices" that compete for the smoker's attention: one that says "I want to *not* smoke anymore," and one that says, "I really want a cigarette right now." Then ask the client to rate the strength of these voices as they apply to them personally. The two ratings can then be used as coordinates to mark the client's location in the *motivational assessment space* diagram on the assessment interview form. Movement within this space can be monitored throughout treatment and can provide an index of shifts in the strength of smoking urges relative to the strength of resolve to become and stay smoke free.

Smoking-related background information

The first two questions pertain to *interests and hobbies* and how they are associated with smoking. This information is important because many of the client's leisure and fun activities will be associated with smoking. Giving up smoking often means losing out (at least temporarily) on important sources of fun and pleasure. For example, a client who regularly goes on fishing trips with a small group of long-time friends, who all are heavy smokers, will experience a sense of loss when considering a switch to fishing alone or finding other, non-smoking companions. Others may enjoy reading and have done so for years while enjoying a cigarette at the same time. The client will need to learn to pursue such activities without smoking, or if that proves too challenging, at least temporarily pursue alternative fun activities. In sum, information on interests and hobbies is instrumental in identifying potential barriers to a smoke-free lifestyle and in designing an individual treatment plan that proactively addresses the risk of leaving a void in terms of pleasurable activities and social connectedness following smoking cessation.

The next two questions ask about *health or medical issues* relevant to smoking and about comorbid substance use other than nicotine. When clients reveal *health conditions*, this is often accompanied by expressions of worry and anxiety (e.g., "what will become of my children?"). The interviewer should use empathic listening here and demonstrate sensitivity and compassion. Sometimes clients do not wish other group members to know about their medical issues. Always clarify what aspects of their medical issue they wish to keep private. Other times, clients are very open about it and talk about it as a particular strong motivator to become smoke free with the help of the group.

If *comorbid problem use of alcohol or other drugs* is present, clients should be advised to seek treatment and be provided with referral information. A special case is the smoking of marijuana. Some clients express a goal of becoming a "non-smoker" but only with respect to cigarettes. They wish to continue smoking marijuana on an occasional or regular basis. Those clients should be advised that the aim of the group is to achieve freedom from all smoking, including smoking marijuana. In our experience, those clients who succeed in cutting down cigarette smoking and becoming smoke free typically report a parallel decline in marijuana use, despite their initial insistence on maintaining the habit.

The next two questions ask about *psychiatric history*. It is not uncommon that individuals presenting for smoking cessation treatment have also received psychological treatments in the past or are concurrently experiencing problems such as depression and anxiety. Many smokers report that smoking helps them to deal with such conditions or other stressors in their life. Because smoking often serves as a "crutch" for these clients to cope with emotional and stressful situations, it is important to identify those links so that these perceived benefits of smoking do not undermine the client's goal of becoming smoke free. Clients should be reassured in the interview that some of the modules of the treatment programs are specifically designed to help clients to manage difficult emotional and stressful situations in alternative ways without resorting to smoking as a coping strategy. As mentioned with other health issues above, always clarify which aspects of a client's emotional or stressful circumstances they wish to keep private from other group members. If appropriate, provide referral information to clients if it appears they could benefit from receiving professional help for their psychological stressors. Difficulty coping on their own with ongoing distress of this nature is often a reason for clients to drop out of smoking cessation treatment, because they lack the strength to take on both at the same time.

The next question asks about *medications* the client is currently taking. Some medications and medical conditions are contraindicated with using pharmacological treatments to help with smoking cessation, such as bupropion or nicotine-replacement products. If a client reports taking medication, advice the client to consult with their prescribing doctor regarding the safety of using pharmacological smoking cessation aids (Chapter 5 has more information on side effects and contraindications of pharmacological treatments).

Carbon monoxide test

A Carbon Monoxide (CO) monitor is a valuable aid in smoking cessation treatment. For the therapist, it can verify that clients are not smoking, and for the client it can serve as a motivational tool. It is very rewarding for clients to observe that cutting down on their cigarette use is accompanied by a decline in their CO reading (in parts per million: COppm). Likewise, it is objective evidence for achieving a tangible health benefit when clients receive confirmation that, after 24 hours of smoking their last cigarette, CO has been eliminated from their body and their reading is comparable to that of non-smokers. There are two client handouts used in conjunction with the CO monitoring. The first is called *Carbon monoxide (CO) monitoring information sheet* and should be given to clients at the time of their first CO testing during the assessment interview. The second is called *Carbon monoxide (CO) feedback chart* and can be used to provide interpretive feedback to clients after each testing of CO levels. Both handouts are in the third part of this chapter, which contains the *Client materials*.

Evaluation of smoker and non-smoker self-concept

Chapter 10 describes the strategies for actively helping clients from day one of the program to shift away from a self-image as a smoker toward a self-image as a non-smoker. At the assessment interview, clients are asked to complete a brief questionnaire to assess quantitatively the relative strength of their self-concept as a smoker and a non-smoker, respectively. The *Smoker and non-smoker self-concept evaluation* form is included in the therapist materials of this chapter. It is very easy to score. To calculate the smoker self-concept score, add items 1, 3, 4, 7, and 9, and divide the sum by 5. To calculate the non-smoker self-concept score, add items 2, 5, 6, and 8, and divide the sum by 4. Each score can range from 0 to 8, with higher scores indicating a stronger self-concept.

General client characteristics relevant to group processes

In addition to collecting assessment information specifically related to symptom presentation, the assessment interview for group treatment also serves to note any individual client features that may be relevant to group processes. We have already noted in the context of taking a medical history that it is important to assess what information about themselves clients are happy to share with the group, and what to keep private. The therapist must use this information skillfully when conducting the group sessions so that no inadvertent disclosures occur that can cause embarrassment and compromise the effectiveness of the group format. Other information relevant to group processes concerns preexisting relationships between group members and interpersonal styles.

It is not uncommon for people to join a smoking cessation group together with a friend, spouse, or work colleague, so that they can provide each other with motivation and support. This can have many benefits. However, it is important for the therapist to be mindful that the dynamics of pairs or subgroups within the group is managed positively and does not "hijack" the agenda to the detriment of the other group members.

With respect to interpersonal characteristics, the assessment interview also reveals who is likely to be very talkative and who may be more shy and reserved in a group context. To get the first group interaction off to a good start, it is best to call initially on group members who appear at ease when communicating, while not being overbearing, and then gently draw in the less-outgoing clients a little later. Conversely, it would not be a good idea to start group interactions with an extremely talkative client, because such a client may command so much attention that less-assertive members may feel discouraged to contribute, and the therapist may have difficulty reining in an overly verbose client before it becomes off-putting to other group members. Thus, taking these individual client features into consideration when planning the group sessions helps to get the group going while ensuring that all group members receive equal attention.

Finally, the personal meanings, circumstances, and events that clients relate during the assessment interview with respect to their struggles to become smoke free provides a wealth of client-generated examples that can be used during treatment to personalize explanations of the treatment rationale, principles, and strategies.

Establishing rapport and a spirit of collaboration

When conducting individual assessments for a group treatment program, collecting the information essential for treatment planning is only one aim. It is also important to prepare the client for the group and start building rapport. Page and Stritzke (2006) recommend covering the following six points when orienting clients for participation in a group.

Enlist clients as informed allies. Tell clients that nicotine addiction is maintained by both behavior and nicotine's effects on the brain. Therefore, treatment involves a combination of strategies that target both – changing behavior and weakening nicotine's hold on the brain.

Offer guidelines about how to participate best in the group. Tell clients that *change comes from doing things differently.* Emphasize that they are expected to take responsibility for putting the strategies they learn into practice. Stress the importance of punctual and regular attendance. Explain that they will get the most out of the group if they participate actively and provide support to fellow group members.

Clarify the format and duration of the program. Remind clients that the group runs for 10 weekly sessions, with one follow-up session about a month after the tenth session. Inform them about the relative timing of initiating behavioral strategies, followed by preparation for "quit day" and nicotine-replacement therapy. Explain that there is important work for them to do *between* sessions with the help of handouts, worksheets, and goal-attainment monitoring materials. Tell them that each two-hour session is divided into two parts, with the first part reviewing client progress, and the second part introducing and practicing change strategies. Clarify who will be running the group. These preparatory steps help to get the ball rolling quickly and allay anticipatory anxiety that may stem from being uncertain about what to expect from the group.

Set ground rules. Less is more! But two rules are essential for groups to function effectively: (a) what occurs in the group remains confidential, and (b) time and attention in the group are shared equally. Explain that clients are free to share their experiences and benefits from the group with others not in the group, but they must not share any identifying information that could be linked to a person, place, or event associated with another member of the group. Encourage them to be active but also to be mindful of the needs of others in the group.

Anticipate frustration and disappointment along the way. Tell clients that the program does not offer quick fixes, but that it offers a proven path to a smoke-free life. Explain that some clients will move along that path quicker than others, and that some setbacks along the way are normal. Reassure clients that the program will help them to view setbacks as opportunities to learn how to do better and succeed the next day.

Instill faith in the program and optimism about the outcome. Tell clients that this program is based on scientific evidence. Reassure them that the principles and strategies used have been shown to work and have helped many smokers to become smoke free. Provide praise for having taking the first step toward a process of change that will lead to a smoke-free lifestyle.

Once you have accumulated your own outcome data from previous groups, you can also use those "local" data to provide further reassurance that clients who fully engage in the program have good success rates.

Progress monitoring and outcome evaluation

For clients to *do things differently*, they need to know what they are *doing*. Progress monitoring tells the client and the therapist what the clients are doing or not doing with respect to working toward their goal to become smoke free. Outcome evaluation tells the client and the therapist to what extent that goal was achieved. Unless the client and therapist collect data on the things clients are supposed to do differently, there is no way of knowing if progress toward goal attainment is being made. Data are the tangible readout for the client to see that their efforts made a difference. They are also the empirical foundation of accountability in practice.

Progress monitoring

It is essential to communicate to clients from the outset (i.e., during the assessment interview) the importance of monitoring. Emphasize how daily and weekly monitoring helps clients to take responsibility for their own change. Explain how monitoring provides important data to track small changes over time. Partial immediate success can be experienced along the way even before reaching the final as yet distant goal of being smoke free. Point out that active participation by clients in ongoing measurement helps to maintain focus on the difficult task at hand and to identify motivational barriers. The above points will be explained again during the first group session when clients are instructed on how to use the *Daily monitoring sheet.*

Progress monitoring is consistent with a low-threshold approach, because goals can be set individually and pursued at different rates in the context of iterative treatment planning. An effective tool to facilitate goal attainment is to illustrate progress through graphing at both the individual and group level. The following examples illustrate four individual progress graphs typically encountered when conducting this treatment program. The graphs are of a type that can track two key outcomes (average daily cigarette intake and weekly CO readings) at the same time. (See *Therapist materials* section for some hints on how to create these graphs by using a few simple steps in a graphing program such as Excel; see Chapter 7 for further information on how to use such graphs in motivational interviewing.)

Figure 2.1 shows the progress profile for patient A. This patient was a very heavy smoker (60 cigarettes/day) prior to the group. Using the change strategies introduced in the first week, she had managed to cut her average

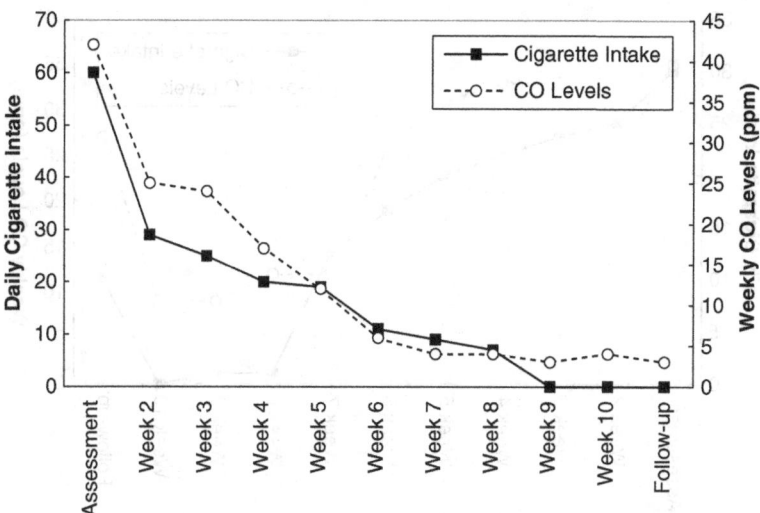

Figure 2.1 Progress profile for patient A with daily cigarette intake and carbon monoxide levels CO, parts per million [ppm].

daily cigarette intake by half (29 cigarettes/day) by the second week, with a further reduction to about 20 cigarettes/day by week 5. Her COppm declined in parallel. Near the end of treatment and at the one-month follow-up she was smoke free and her COppm was comparable to that of a non-smoker.

Patient B (Figure 2.2) also showed a steady decline from heavy smoking (30 cigarettes/day) prior to treatment to only sporadic smoking in weeks 8 and 9, and no cigarette intake in the final week of the program. This patient had relapsed to smoking around 12 cigarettes/day at follow-up. Note that the self-reported decline in number of cigarettes smoked early in treatment was not initially matched by a decline in CO level. There could be several reasons why the COppm appear higher than they should be based on the self-report data. One is that some smokers will compensate for smoking fewer cigarettes by trying to get more out of each cigarette (Benowitz *et al.*, 1986). For example, they draw harder on the cigarettes, inhale deeper by holding the smoke longer in their lungs before exhaling, and smoke the cigarette all the way down to the filter. Another possibility is that this client was not telling the truth when reporting his level of daily cigarette intake. Yet another possibility is that this person was exposed to other sources of CO pollution in the environment in addition to his smoking. It is important to consider these alternative explanations when discussing such a profile with a client. If the client was not telling the truth, the CO readings may help to prompt more honest reporting and renewed efforts to engage in the change strategies. In this particular case, the client

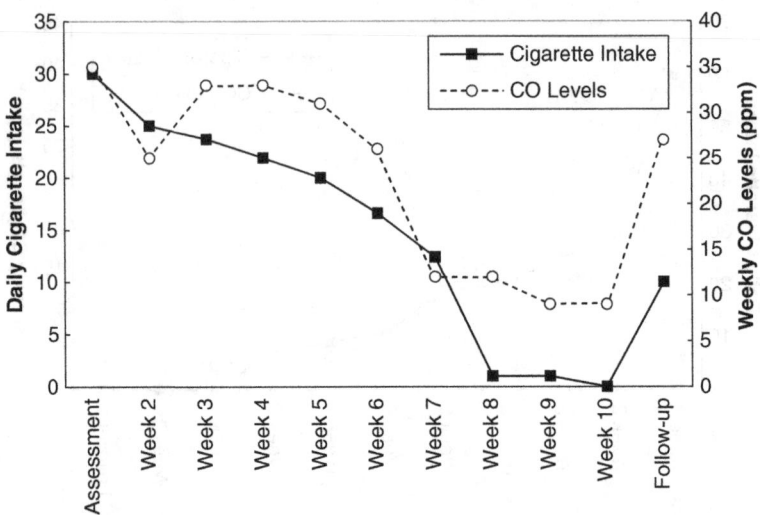

Figure 2.2 Progress profile for patient B with daily cigarette intake and carbon monoxide levels CO, parts per million [ppm].

was a taxi driver who spent many hours each day exposed to car exhaust fumes in traffic and when waiting in taxi pick-up areas. This could explain his higher than expected COppm.

The profile of patient C (Figure 2.3) shows how a steep decline in average daily cigarette intake was accompanied by an equally steep decline in CO levels. This patient had temporarily dropped out of the group program for health reasons, but after rejoining made up for lost time and achieved reduction in daily smoking and smoke free status in a much less gradual fashion than patients A and B. Note that the sharp declining slope of the self-reported cigarette use was confirmed by the similarly sharp drop in the slope of the COppm values.

Patient D (Figure 2.4) reported only a light level of smoking (6 cigarettes/day) at the time of assessment. The corresponding COppm reading was, therefore, at the low end of the range expected for a light smoker (see *Carbon monoxide (CO) feedback chart* on p. 44). This patient quit smoking after the assessment interview and before the first group session. He wanted to attend the group nonetheless to prevent him from relapsing. Consequently, starting from week 1, his COppm readings were consistently well within the range (<10) expected for a non-smoker, except in week 5. On the day of the CO testing in week 5 and the day prior to it, there had been a large forest fire near the patient's home, with resultant heavy smoke pollution in this area. Therefore, similar to patient B's profile, which reflected chronic workplace exposure to higher than normal levels of CO in the environment,

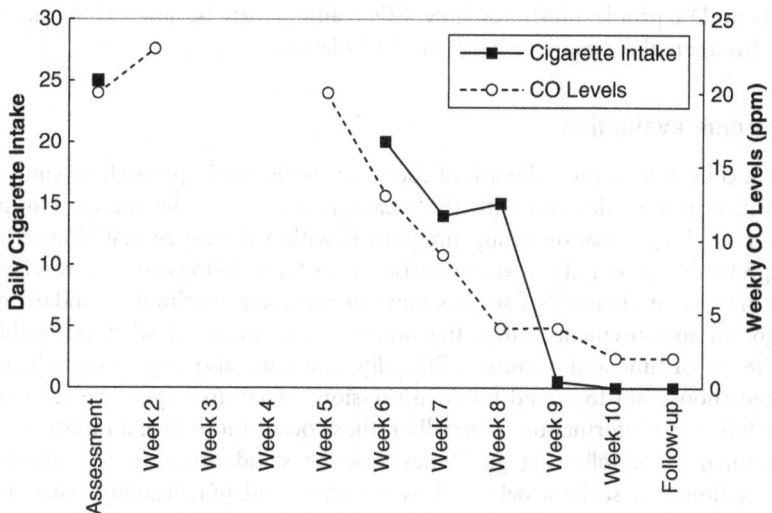

Figure 2.3 Progress profile for patient C with daily cigarette intake and carbon monoxide levels CO, parts per million [ppm].

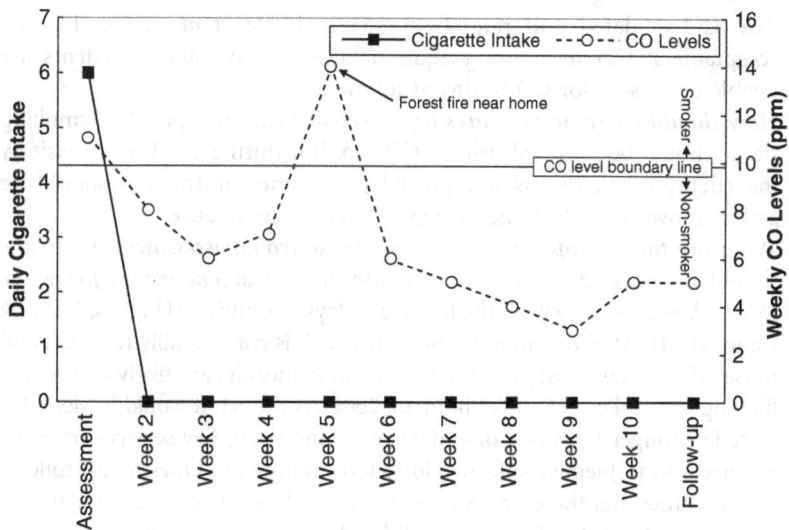

Figure 2.4 Progress profile for patient D with daily cigarette intake and carbon monoxide levels CO, parts per million [ppm].

patient D's profile illustrates how CO readings can be affected by acute environmental exposure to heightened CO levels.

Outcome evaluation

Data collection is the hallmark of the science-informed approach to clinical practice. It provides you with the means to show that the success rate of your smoking cessation group program is within the range that should be expected based on published comparison rates for smoking cessation services. In practice, evaluation of success aims to achieve a minimum standard of rigor in measurement within the practical constraints of what is feasible in terms of time and resources. Ethically, one must also respect that clients often choose not to attend follow-up sessions or fail to respond to requests for follow-up information, especially if those occur more than a month after treatment. The following guidelines describe standards of good outcome evaluation that strike a balance between rigor and practicability. They are largely consistent with "The Russell Standard (Clinical)" (West, 2005), which clarifies monitoring requirements set out by the health authorities in the UK (Department of Health, 2001).

1 *What are the key outcome measures?* Self-reported number of cigarettes smoked combined with a CO reading provide the most reliable and valid index of smoking status. Self-reported quit rates alone tend to be higher than CO-validated quit rates by 14–51% (Judge *et al.*, 2005), but are acceptable if CO monitoring equipment is not available or clients are unable to present for CO testing at follow-up.

2 *How should outcome measures be collected?* Whenever possible, smoking status should be recorded using a CO monitor during a follow-up visit by the client. When this is not possible, outcome information should be gathered over the telephone or by written correspondence.

3 *What are the appropriate time points for outcome assessment?* Outcome should be assessed at the *end of treatment* and at *one-month follow-up*. Most relapses occur within the first eight days of quitting (Hughes, Keely, & Naud, 2004). After one month, the relapse risk is considerably reduced, and those who remain abstinent for two to three months are likely to become lifelong ex-smokers (West & Shiffman, 2004). Although it would be desirable to collect longer-term outcome data (e.g., one year), few services have the resources to implement effective long-term follow-up. One-month follow-up outcomes are, therefore, a reasonably good estimate of treatment success, especially if they have been validated by CO assessment.

4 *What are the criteria for counting a treated smoker as a successful quitter?* A smoker who (a) reports to have been smoke free for a period of four weeks after his or her designated quit date, and (b) shows expired-air CO readings of less than 10ppm four weeks after the quit date (minus three

days or plus two weeks), can be counted as a successful quitter. Some monitoring guidelines may additionally require that smoke-free clients in the two weeks prior to follow-up assessment have not smoked even a single puff on a cigarette.

5 *Who should be counted in determining who succeeded and who did not?* Smokers who attended the assessment session and the first session of the treatment program, but failed to attend thereafter, are not included in the count. They cannot be regarded as "treated smokers" because they never did engage with the treatment program. That is, once the change strategies were introduced in the first session and the responsibility for applying these strategies toward goal attainment on a daily basis subsequent to that session had been placed firmly in the clients' hands, these "drop-outs" had elected to opt out of treatment before getting started.

6 *How is the success rate calculated?* The four-week, CO-verified success rate as a percentage is calculated by dividing the number of "successful quitters" by the number of "treated smokers" and then multiplying it by 100. For example, consider a group that started out with 12 members who had attended the pre-group assessment interview. Two of the people who had been assessed did not show up for the first or any subsequent group session, and one married couple who had joined the group together dropped out after the first treatment session. Therefore, regardless of whether the eight remaining members completed the program or dropped out at a later time, all eight are counted as "treated smokers." If four of them were smoke free four weeks after their designated quit date validated by expired-air CO readings, the success rate would be $[(4/8) \times 100] = 50\%$. Group members for whom follow-up data are not available are assumed to be smokers.

7 *What is the benchmark for evaluating success?* The outcomes achieved for any given group within a local treatment setting can be compared with success rates of (a) *untreated smokers* who quit on their own and (b) *treated smokers* who quit with the help of similar smoking cessation services (i.e., those combining cognitive–behavioral strategies with pharmacotherapies). Table 2.1 lists short-term and long-term CO-validated cessation rates that can be expected for untreated and treated smokers, and against which the success rates achieved at a local treatment service can be compared. Ideally, one-month follow-up outcomes of a smoking cessation group should exceed those achieved by smokers quitting on their own (i.e., >28%) and should be comparable to the average success rates published in the litera-ture for similar cessation services (i.e., ≥53%). However, when using these published rates as a benchmark for success, one must be mindful of two things. First, there is considerable variability in cessation rates reported across different smoking cessation services, with four-week cessation rates varying from 22% to 79% (Bauld *et al.*, 2003). Second, even though cessation rates at the low end of this continuum may be no better than those of

Table 2.1. Short-term and long-term carbon monoxide-validated smoking cessation rates[a]

	Smoking cessation rates at follow-up (%)	
	One month	12 months
Untreated smokers	15–28[1]	2–7[2]
Treated smokers	53[3]	15[4]

Note:
[a]Self-reported rates that are not validated by carbon monoxide measurements, on average, tend to exceed those listed in this table.
Sources: 1. Hughes *et al.*, (2004); 2. Cohen *et al.*, (1989); 3. Judge *et al.*, (2005); 4. Ferguson *et al.*, (2005).

smokers quitting on their own, they still represent clinically significant improvements and hence value for money from the point of view of population health (West, 2007).

8 *Is long-term abstinence the only valid indicator of success?* Although long-term abstinence can be regarded as the gold standard for evaluating smoking cessation interventions, it is by no means the only meaningful outcome measure. Among heavy smokers (15+cigarettes/day), smoking reduction by more than 50% has significant health benefits (Bollinger *et al.*, 2002; Godtfredsen *et al.*, 2005), reduces toxin intake (Wennike *et al.*, 2003), and increases the likelihood of becoming smoke free at future cessation attempts (Hughes, 2000; Hyland *et al.*, 2005). Low-rate and occasional smokers are three times more likely to quit smoking than regular daily smokers (Zhu *et al.*, 2003). However, because reductions in daily cigarette intake may be accompanied by compensatory smoking, it is essential that these reductions are validated by CO assessment. That is, the decrease in CO levels should be proportional to the amount of reduction in cigarette intake. If compensatory smoking does occur, the health benefits of reducing intake are questionable (see Box 2.1).

A brief *Outcome evaluation form* is included in the *Therapist materials* section of this chapter. This form can be used at the end of treatment and at follow-up to record essential outcome information. The first question determines current smoking status. If the client is not smoke free, current level of smoking is assessed in the second question, and then the smoker is directed to question 10 to assess current level of ambivalence toward change. This information can be useful in advising unsuccessful group members on treatment options for further quit attempts. If clients are smoke free, they skip the second question and complete the remainder of the evaluation form. Question 3 records the designated quit day, and in question 4 the current CO reading is entered (Note: the CO reading can already be entered into the form by the person administering the CO test before asking the client to complete the remainder of the form). Question 6 determines if the client has had a single puff on a cigarette in the past two weeks, and questions 7 and 8 record if the client used any pharmacological aids. Question 9 assesses the level of any potential withdrawal distress experienced by the client. That is, Questions 7 to 10 try to identify the degree of withdrawal distress and the strength of residual motivational ambivalence, which provides an estimate of the continuing effort required by the client to successfully manage relapse risk.

Tips for working with individuals

The same structured interview template can be used whether clients are assessed for individual or group interventions. The primary aims of the assessment interview are identical whether group or individual interventions are planned:

- gathering information about the individual's smoking history and other core dimensions relevant to smoking cessation (aim 1)
- developing a treatment plan by conceptualizing which individual client characteristics are optimally addressed by which components of the treatment program (aim 3a)
- establishing rapport and a spirit of collaboration (aim 4)
- establishing a baseline of critical change variables against which progress and outcomes can be evaluated (aim 5).

Two of the aims of the assessment protocol described in this chapter are not relevant for individual interventions and, therefore, it simplifies the assessment protocol. There is obviously no need to identify client characteristics and circumstances that may either facilitate or potentially hinder group processes (aim 2). Likewise, one does not need to assess how the client's individual smoking history or motivations and circumstances of becoming smoke free could best be brought into play in capitalizing on group processes when engaging clients in the different treatment components (aim 3b). As there is no need for the assessment information to inform group processes or to prepare the individual client during the assessment interview for a group-based intervention, this simplifies the assessment process. Although the information gathered is the same for individual and group interventions, what one does with the information for treatment planning is less complex for individual interventions, as the intervention plan is tailored only to the individual's situation.

The following parts of the *Therapist guidelines* are either not relevant or can be adapted for individual interventions.

Tips (cont.)

- The section *General client characteristics relevant to group processes* can be ignored.
- Of the bulleted points in the section *Establishing rapport and a spirit of collaboration*, the first point (enlist clients as informed allies) and the last point (instill faith in the program and optimism about the outcome) also apply to individual interventions. Three of the points (offering guidelines about how to participate, clarifying format and duration of the program, and anticipating frustration and disappointment along the way) still apply but need to be focused on the individual rather than group context. The one point about setting ground rules can be ignored.
- Within the *Outcome evaluation* section, outcome data should still be reported cumulatively for a given reporting period and number of clients treated within that period. Of course, if the intervention is not group based, the additional, useful information on success rates for a given group, or average success rates across different groups, cannot be computed.

THERAPIST MATERIALS

The following materials are given.
1 Assessment interview form for smoking cessation group
2 Fagerström test for nicotine dependence (FTND)
3 Smoker and non-smoker self-concept evaluation form
4 Hints on how to create progress graphs in Excel
5 Outcome evaluation form.

Assessment interview form for smoking cessation group

INTRODUCTION

- *Briefly state the parameters of confidentiality in accordance with the policies of your practice or service agency.*
- *Tell the client*: "The aim of the interview is to collect information about your smoking history and your desire to become smoke free, and also to provide you with information about the group and what you can do to get the most out of the treatment program."
- *Tell the client*: "It is important that you are as honest as possible so that we can make the group as effective for you as possible."

REFERRAL INFORMATION

With the next two questions, find out what the client's reasons are for coming to the group, and whether they are self-generated or stem from outside influences. Identify any specific events that influenced the person's decision to come at this time.

- What brings you here now?

  _____
  _____
  _____
  _____

- What do you hope to achieve by coming to the group?

  _____
  _____
  _____
  _____

PATTERN AND CONTEXT OF CIGARETTE SMOKING

- When did you start smoking?

  _____

- What prompted you to start smoking?

  _____
  _____
  _____

- How many cigarettes do you smoke per day?

  _____

- How much money do you spend on cigarettes per day?

  _____

- What pack size do you buy?

  _____

- What is the nicotine level of the cigarettes you smoke?

  _____

- How soon after you wake up do you smoke your first cigarette?

  _____

- Have you experienced any withdrawal symptoms in the past?
  Yes ☐   No ☐
- (*If yes*) What were they, and how bad did they get?

  _____

  _____

  _____

  _____

- What was your longest time without a cigarette in the last week?

  _____

- What was your longest time without a cigarette in the last year?

  _____

- Have you ever tried to quit smoking in the past?
  Yes ☐   No ☐
- Have you ever used nicotine-replacement treatment in the past?
  Yes ☐   No ☐
- Have you ever used Zyban (bupropion) in the past?
  Yes ☐   No ☐
- How long ago was your last attempt to quit smoking?

  _____

- For how long did you manage to stay smoke free after quitting in the past?

  _____

  _____

  _____

- When you managed to quit smoking for a while, what helped?

  _____

  _____

  _____

- For how long have you been smoking at the current level?

  _____

MOTIVATION FOR CHANGE AND POTENTIAL BARRIERS TO CHANGE

- How likely do you think it is that you will be a non-smoker in six months time, on a scale from 1 (not likely) to 10 (very likely)?

1	2	3	4	5	6	7	8	9	10
Not likely									Very likely

Ask for the reasons why the client gave the particular rating s/he gave. (e.g., "Why did you rate the likelihood of being a non-smoker in six months a '6' rather than a '10'?")

_____

_____

_____

_____

- How ready are you to change and become a non-smoker, on a scale from 1 (low readiness to change) to 10 (high readiness to change)?

_____

1	2	3	4	5	6	7	8	9	10

Low readiness   High readiness

- Are there certain occasions where you feel it is particularly difficult not to have a cigarette?

_____

_____

_____

_____

_____

- Are there certain occasions where you find it easier to abstain from smoking?

_____

_____

_____

_____

- Are you currently living with anyone that smokes?
  Yes ☐   No ☐
  (*If yes*) What is their attitude towards smoking/quitting?

_____

_____

_____

_____

- Are there people that support your decision to quit?
  Yes ☐   No ☐
  (*If yes*) Who are they?

_____

_____

_____

_____

Now assess the level of ambivalence toward change.

- *First explain:* "Often people who want to quit smoking have two voices in their head, one that says 'I want to not smoke anymore', and another that says 'I really want a cigarette right now'."
- *Then ask:* "Please rate how strong each one of those two voices was for you personally in the last 24 hours, on a scale from 0 (very weak) to 8 (very strong)."
- How strong was the voice saying "I want to not smoke anymore?"

0	1	2	3	4	5	6	7	8
Very weak							Very strong	

- How strong was the voice saying "I really want a cigarette right now?"

0	1	2	3	4	5	6	7	8
Very weak							Very strong	

Use the above ratings as coordinates and mark client's location in the following diagram:

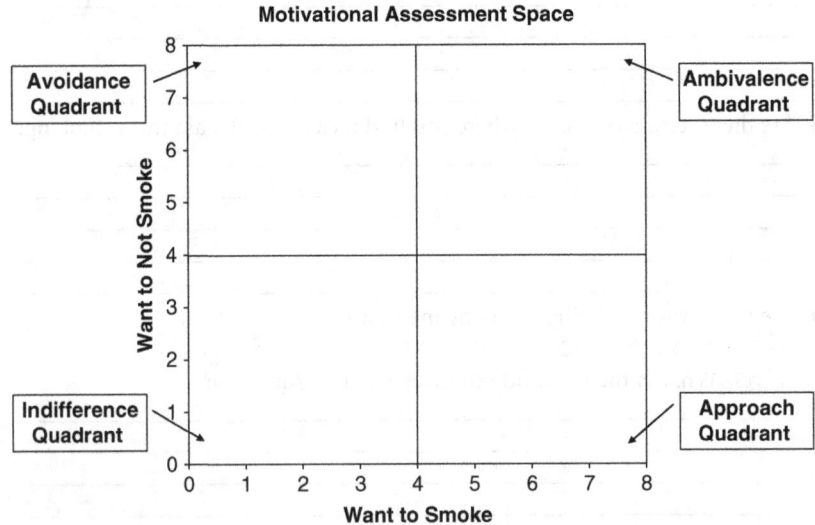

SMOKING-RELATED BACKGROUND INFORMATION

Interests and hobbies:
- What are your interests and hobbies?

_____
_____
_____
_____

- How are these associated with smoking? Can you do these activities without having a cigarette?

_____

_____

_____

_____

Health and medical history, particularly with regard to smoking:

- Have you had any medical or health conditions related to your smoking?
  Yes ☐   No ☐

_____

_____

_____

_____

- Do you drink alcohol or use drugs that are not prescribed by a doctor?
  Yes ☐   No ☐

_____

_____

_____

_____

Psychiatric history:

- Have you had any previous psychotherapy or counseling?
  Yes ☐   No ☐
  (*If yes*) When? What did you seek help for? Where?

_____

_____

_____

_____

- Are you currently experiencing any emotional difficulties or stressors?
  Yes ☐   No ☐

_____

_____

_____

_____

Medications:
- Are you currently taking any medications?
  Yes ☐   No ☐
  (*If yes*) Type   Dose

_____

_____

_____

_____
_____
_____
_____

CARBON MONOXIDE (CO) TEST

Administer CO monitor and record:

* Date   _____ (dd/mm/yy)

* Time since last cigarette   _____ (minutes)

  CO (ppm) reading   _____ (COppm)

Fagerström Test for Nicotine Dependence

These questions help you to determine how dependent you are on your cigarettes.
Please tick the box next to the answers that best describe your smoking behavior.

• How soon after you wake up do you smoke your first cigarette?	☐ Within 5 minutes	3
	☐ 6–30 minutes	2
	☐ More than 30 minutes	1
• Do you find it difficult to refrain from smoking in places where smoking is not permitted?	☐ Yes	1
	☐ No	0
• Which cigarette would you hate most to give up?	☐ The first one in the morning	1
	☐ Others	0
• How many cigarettes per day do you usually smoke?	☐ 10 or less	0
	☐ 11–20	1
	☐ 21–30	2
	☐ 31 or more	3
• Do you smoke more frequently during the first hours after waking then during the rest of the day?	☐ Yes	1
	☐ No	0
• Do you smoke if you are so ill that you are in bed most of the day?	☐ Yes	1
	☐ No	0

Total score (max. = 10) ☐

Note:
(Permission to reproduce the Fagerström Test for Nicotine Dependence (Heatherton *et al.*, 1991) for this manual granted by Blackwell Publishing.)

Smoker and non-smoker self-concept evaluation

This questionnaire relates to your self-image as a *smoker* and a *non-smoker* at this moment in time. Please indicate how much you agree with the statements below by circling the number corresponding most closely to your self-image RIGHT NOW. Your answers may range from AGREE NOT AT ALL (0) with the statement to AGREE VERY STRONGLY (8) with the statement.

I AGREE WITH THIS STATEMENT...

	not at all							very strongly
1 Smoking is part of my self-image	0 1 2 3 4 5 6 7 8
2 It is easy to imagine myself as a non-smoker	0 1 2 3 4 5 6 7 8
3 Smoking is part of "who I am"	0 1 2 3 4 5 6 7 8
4 Smoking is a large part of my daily life	0 1 2 3 4 5 6 7 8
5 I am comfortable with the idea of being a non-smoker	0 1 2 3 4 5 6 7 8
6 Not Smoking is "like me"	0 1 2 3 4 5 6 7 8
7 Smoking is part of my personality	0 1 2 3 4 5 6 7 8
8 I am able to see myself as a non-smoker	0 1 2 3 4 5 6 7 8
9 Others view smoking as part of my personality	0 1 2 3 4 5 6 7 8

(Adapted from Shadel & Mermelstein, 1996.)

Hints on how to create progress graphs in Excel

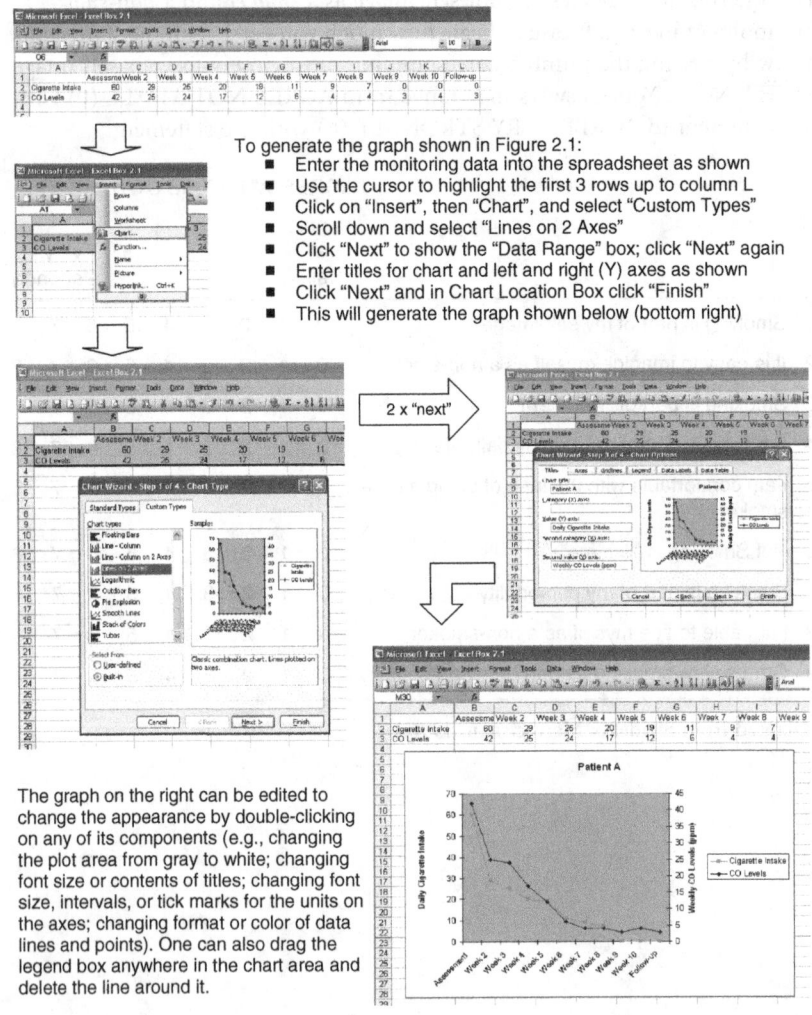

To generate the graph shown in Figure 2.1:
- Enter the monitoring data into the spreadsheet as shown
- Use the cursor to highlight the first 3 rows up to column L
- Click on "Insert", then "Chart", and select "Custom Types"
- Scroll down and select "Lines on 2 Axes"
- Click "Next" to show the "Data Range" box; click "Next" again
- Enter titles for chart and left and right (Y) axes as shown
- Click "Next" and in Chart Location Box click "Finish"
- This will generate the graph shown below (bottom right)

The graph on the right can be edited to change the appearance by double-clicking on any of its components (e.g., changing the plot area from gray to white; changing font size or contents of titles; changing font size, intervals, or tick marks for the units on the axes; changing format or color of data lines and points). One can also drag the legend box anywhere in the chart area and delete the line around it.

Outcome evaluation form

Client ID: _____   Date: ____/____/____

1 Are you smoke free now?
  Yes □   No □
  If yes, go to question 3
  If no, go to question 2

2 How many cigarettes do you smoke per day?

  _____

  Now go to question 10

3 When was your designated quit date?
  _____/_____/_____
  (dd)   (mm)   (yyyy)

4 What is your current carbon monoxide (CO) test reading?
  _____ (COppm)

5 For how many days have you been smoke free?

  _____

6 Have you had a single puff on a cigarette in the past two weeks?
  Yes □   No □

7 Did you use nicotine-replacement products (e.g., patches)?
  Yes □   No □

8 Did you use Zyban (bupropion)?
  Yes □   No □

9 Have you experienced any withdrawal symptoms?
  Yes □   No □

  If yes
  How bad did they get *at their worst?*
  not too bad □   bad □   extremely bad □

  How are they *now?*
  gone □   not too bad □   bad □   extremely bad □

10 Often people who want to quit smoking or who have recently become
   smoke free have two voices in their head, one that says *"I want to not
   smoke anymore,"* and another that says *"I really want a cigarette right now."*
   Please rate how strong each one of those two voices was for you personally
   in the last 24 hours, on a scale from 0 (very weak) to 8 (very strong)

(a) How strong was the voice saying *"I want to not smoke anymore?"*

| 0 | 1 | 2 | 3 | 4 | 5 | 6 | 7 | 8 |

Very weak   Very strong

(b) How strong was the voice saying *"I really want a cigarette right now?"*

| 0 | 1 | 2 | 3 | 4 | 5 | 6 | 7 | 8 |

Very weak   Very strong

CLIENT MATERIALS

1 Carbon monoxide (CO) monitoring information sheet
2 Carbon monoxide (CO) feedback chart

Carbon monoxide (CO) monitoring information sheet

What is carbon monoxide or CO?

Carbon monoxide is a poisonous gas that can be found in polluted air, car exhaust fumes, and in tobacco smoke. It is absorbed into the blood from the lungs and is a rough indicator of how much a smoker has smoked within the past 24 hours.

What does the CO monitor measure?

When you exhale into the CO monitor, it measures the amount of CO in your expired air. The amount of CO in the air exhaled from your lungs gives an indication of how much CO is in your blood.

How does CO harm your body?

CO takes the place of oxygen in your red blood cells. Smokers can have between 2 and 20% of the normal oxygen carried in their blood replaced by CO. Also, CO reduces the release of oxygen. The body needs oxygen to live, and CO deprives the body of oxygen.

What are the consequences of high CO levels in your blood?

To make up for the shortage of oxygen in your blood, your body needs to work harder with less fuel. This is damaging to your health because:

- the smoker's heart beats faster trying to get enough oxygen to the body
- the smoker's heart gets less oxygen, which can damage heart muscles and lead to sudden death
- because there is little extra oxygen to spare, the smoker gets easily breathless when putting extra demand on the body by any kind of exercise
- the reduced level of oxygen can cause the lining of smoker's arteries to weaken, allowing more cholesterol in, which, in turn, causes fatty build up and increases the risk of circulation problems, heart attack, and stroke.

What is the good news?

While you are still smoking, your CO readings will be fairly high. But once you have smoked your last cigarette, the CO level in your blood falls almost immediately. After a couple of days, your CO readings will be the same as that of a non-smoker. Your blood will carry more oxygen! This will give you more energy, better circulation, and greater concentration.

What do I need to do when taking the CO test?

It's simple! Take a deep breath and hold it for 15 seconds. Then blow into the CO monitor. Blow out completely. Enter the date and your COppm reading in your CO feedback chart. The COppm reading is the amount of CO in your exhaled breath. The COHb(%) column tells you how much CO is in your blood. COHb(%) means the percentage of red blood cells or hemoglobin (Hb) that is carrying CO instead of oxygen. For example, if your COppm reading is 40, then 7% of your red blood cells are carrying CO.

Carbon monoxide (CO) feedback chart

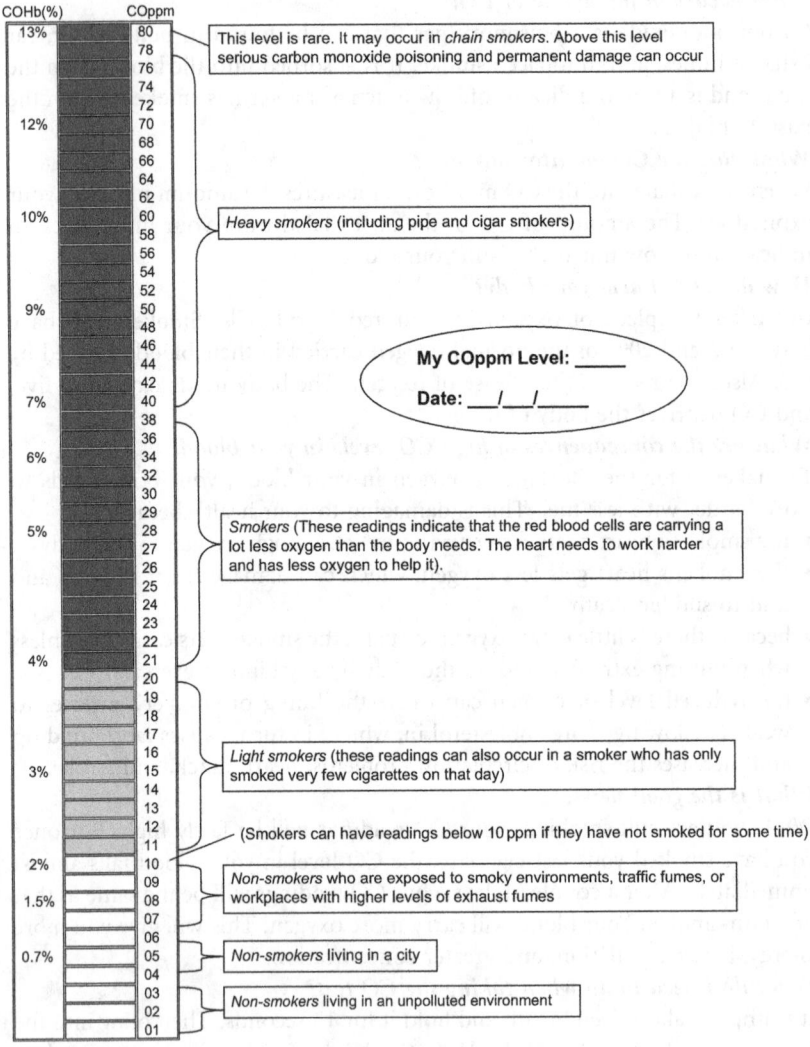

COHb(%)   COppm

13% | 80 — This level is rare. It may occur in *chain smokers*. Above this level serious carbon monoxide poisoning and permanent damage can occur (78, 76, 74, 72)

12% | 70 (68, 66, 64, 62)

10% | 60 — *Heavy smokers* (including pipe and cigar smokers) (58, 56, 54, 52)

9% | 50 (48, 46, 44, 42)

My COppm Level: _____

Date: ___/___/_____

7% | 40 (38, 36)

6% | 34 (32, 30)

5% | 29, 28, 27, 26 — *Smokers* (These readings indicate that the red blood cells are carrying a lot less oxygen than the body needs. The heart needs to work harder and has less oxygen to help it). (25, 24, 23, 22)

4% | 21 (20, 19, 18, 17)

3% | 16, 15, 14 — *Light smokers* (these readings can also occur in a smoker who has only smoked very few cigarettes on that day) (13)

12, 11 — (Smokers can have readings below 10 ppm if they have not smoked for some time)

2% | 10, 09 — *Non-smokers* who are exposed to smoky environments, traffic fumes, or workplaces with higher levels of exhaust fumes

1.5% | 08, 07, 06

0.7% | 05 — *Non-smokers* living in a city (04)

03, 02 — *Non-smokers* living in an unpolluted environment (01)

(Adapted from Smokerlyzers product information, Bedfont Scientific Ltd., 2002.)

Starting the change process

THERAPIST GUIDELINES

Aims

1 Facilitate relationships that are helpful for change
2 Establish guidelines for a successful program and promote group cohesion
3 Explain the nature of nicotine addiction and how our understanding of the mechanisms underlying this addiction provides the rationale for the treatment program
4 Discuss "becoming smoke-free day"
5 Illustrate behavioral component of smoking routines and commence behavioral change strategies
6 Promote self-image as a non-smoker and end on a positive note.

Facilitate helpful relationships

The positive working relationship established in the initial assessment session needs to be strengthened. Congratulate and encourage group members for taking the step to come along to the first session, and be supportive of the journey they are about to embark on. It is important to emphasize a collaborative approach to the smoking cessation program.

Establish guidelines and promote group cohesion

Discuss with group members that one of the benefits of the program is that the group format is like a "buddy system" on a bigger scale, and that they have one another and yourselves, the therapists, to help them on the journey to becoming smoke free and to draw on one another's experiences. Point out that in order to achieve this, there will need to be guidelines for the group so that everyone will feel comfortable with discussing what is happening in their lives and how these events impact on smoking behaviors. Important guidelines include confidentiality, being respectful and non-judgemental of others' situations, allowing others equal time during the sessions, and keeping focused on the aims of the session.

Explain the nature of nicotine addiction and its relation to the treatment program

Discuss the nature of smoking addiction as having both chemical and behavioral components, with both components being very powerful. Explain to group members that while the program aims to help them to break both the chemical and the behavioral addictions, these will be addressed one step at a time (behavioral first then chemical), because doing both at the same time will likely induce more stress than addressing one followed by the other.

Discuss setting the "becoming smoke-free day"

The group members are likely to be expecting the therapists to tell them to stop smoking as of the first session (we often have clients who admit that they smoked "like chimneys" in the hours leading up to the first session so that nothing would "go to waste"). Instead, emphasize the low-threshold approach to change where there is no pressure to set a date immediately by which to be smoke free. The intention is to give group members a chance to be successful at learning some skills that will help them to become and remain smoke free when they are ready. Advise clients that this date will preferably occur just prior to or around the middle of the program. This is because the skills involved in *remaining* smoke free are somewhat different to those involved in *becoming* smoke free, and it is important to allow clients sufficient time after "quit day" to practice their skills at remaining smoke free. Focus on gradually cutting down the number of cigarettes smoked over the weeks on the way to becoming smoke free. Also, phrase quitting in terms of gains rather than losses (i.e., "becoming smoke free" rather than "giving up smoking").

Illustrate the behavioral component of smoking routines and commence behavioral change strategies

Conduct an exercise to demonstrate to clients how powerful the behavioral component of the smoking addiction can be. Ask group members to think about how many times in their lives they have lit a cigarette (how many times they smoke in a day multiplied by the number of days in a year and the the number of years they have been smoking). Do this exercise with them so they gain an idea of the approximate number of times they have lit a cigarette in a lifetime. For example, someone who has smoked about eight cigarettes a day for the past 15 years would have smoked about 43 800 cigarettes, repeating the same action every time they lit up each of those cigarettes.

Pose questions to the group members designed to prompt them to think about the impact of the behavioral addiction. For instance, if someone always has a cigarette after dinner, ask what happens if he/she had two cigarettes *immediately before* dinner – the rationale underlying this being that if smoking was purely a chemical addiction, the chemical addiction should still be satiated right after dinner. If, however, they still have the cigarette, it is because they are used to the habit of having a cigarette after dinner (i.e., having first dinner and then a cigarette have become two activities that are strongly linked).

Use this as a lead-in to introducing the need for behavioral change within the smoking cessation program. Emphasize that, over time, certain cues have become powerfully linked with smoking (e.g., a particular coffee mug used to drink coffee while having an afternoon cigarette). Also, the particular sequence of events leading up to having the first puff of each cigarette is likely to have been repeated so often that it is a very well rehearsed sequence, much like driving. Emphasize that the key to breaking the behavioral habit is to *vary* the smoking routine according to *when, how,* and *where.* Thus, encourage clients to vary where they smoke, vary when they smoke (including the order of the sequence of events leading up to the first puff), and also to vary how they smoke (e.g., smoke with the opposite hand). To help group members to identify how they can break down their individual smoking routines, go through the diagram on *How to change your smoking routine* in the client handout. Then elicit examples of smoking routines from the group so that clients can better grasp this concept in the context of their own day-to-day lives.

Promote self-image as a non-smoker

The first session is likely to be a bit overwhelming for clients, with lots of information to take in and also having to commence change straight away. Make it a point again to congratulate group members for undertaking the journey to become smoke free. Finally, build on the momentum that group members typically experience after coming along to the group by finishing off the session with the imagery exercise *From Smoke City to Fresh Hills.* This exercise is adapted from Marlatt & Gordon (1985) and is designed to help clients to learn to visualize themselves as non smokers: to help them develop a different identity. At the end of this, invite group members to relate the imagery exercise to their own personal circumstances to be shared with everyone at the next group session. Emphasize that there will be temptations along the journey, but that they will learn the skills to weather those temptations successfully and stay smoke free.

Tips for working with individuals

The first aim of this module is to facilitate a collaborative relationship with clients at the start of the program and this is, of course, also important during a one-on-one intervention. However, in the one-on-one context, there is no need to balance individual attention across a number of clients as in group interventions. The second aim of establishing guidelines for group interactions and promoting group cohesion are not relevant when working with individuals. The remaining four aims all apply equally to group and individual interventions. The primary adaptation to working with individual clients is that the exercises to illustrate the behavioral components of smoking routines will be based on the examples provided by the one client rather than on the collective contribution from several clients covering a range of different circumstances.

Likewise, with respect to the client handouts, only minimal adaptations are required. For the most part, an individual client can simply be instructed to ignore any references to interactions with other group members and apply the material directly to themselves. In the first handout, there is a brief section that introduces the group guidelines and aims to reassure group clients who may feel a bit awkward in a group context. This section could be omitted from the handout if used with an individual client.

CLIENT MATERIALS

1 Now that you have decided to become smoke free, what's next?
2 Understanding the nature of nicotine addiction: the chemical addiction and the behavioral addiction
3 Making change happen
4 It's time to start doing things differently!
5 When to set your "becoming smoke free day"
6 From Smoke City to Fresh Hills.

Now that you have decided to become smoke free, what's next?

Congratulations on deciding to become smoke free! We're glad you have taken this important step to a better way of life. We are here to provide you with the skills to stay smoke free and to support you in your travels from being a smoker to becoming a non-smoker. So, if you have any questions along the way, please do not hesitate to ask us.

You have taken a big step in joining the program – we want *you* to recognize how big this step is as well. Make sure you congratulate yourself for making it this far – it shows that you are motivated to improve the quality of your life. Coming along today, however, is only the first step. To successfully make and maintain changes, it is important to keep the motivation up and come along every week. In doing so, you will learn all the strategies that have been proven to be helpful in becoming smoke free. It also means that we can develop a supportive network in the group to help everyone support each other through this challenging journey.

By coming along to the sessions, you will learn skills that help you become and remain smoke free. However, it takes *you* to put those skills into place. That's right, we want you to take control of the changes and be active in doing all the things that bring about change! In this way, you will be able to see the effect you can have in controlling this addiction. The more time and effort you put into actively changing, the easier it will be to become and remain smoke free. Remember, we only see you for a very small part of the week – it is up to you to make the changes between the group sessions. We are here to help you with any difficulties you are experiencing, and also to hear about your successes.

Although we are here to guide and help you, we also think that the support of your fellow group members is important. We understand that a group setting may feel a bit awkward at first for some, and one way to address this is by introducing some group guidelines. A few simple guidelines that make it easier for everyone to feel comfortable in groups like this are:
1 Keep information you learn about others confidential
2 Respect everyone's unique circumstances
3 Allow others equal time
4 Stay focused on the task at hand.

Understanding the nature of nicotine addiction

Giving up smoking is difficult. Remaining smoke free is even more difficult. The reason for the difficulty is that, when moving through the steps of becoming smoke free, you are beating not just one but two "addictions."

The chemical addiction

The first addiction is a chemical one. Nicotine is a powerfully addictive chemical. Nicotine stimulates a part of the brain called the dopamine system. This system is also known as the "reward" pathway and provides the experience of pleasure or a "rush" you feel when you smoke a cigarette. Nicotine is an extremely powerful drug: it takes just a few seconds after inhalation for 90% of the nicotine in the lungs to reach the brain.

The behavioral addiction

Smoking is not just about the chemical addiction. There is also a behavioral component. For instance, if you normally smoke one cigarette each hour but smoke four per hour while socializing with friends in a pub or at a party, then you are not reaching for those cigarettes because of the chemical addiction but rather because you have developed a habit of smoking more cigarettes when having a good time with friends. The behavioral addiction comes about through smoking more in certain situations. This leads to the development of a habit that is difficult to break.

Think of the number of times that you have lit a cigarette in your life. That's an amazing number of opportunities to learn that cigarettes are a part of your everyday functioning! For a regular smoker who smokes 25 cigarettes a day, cigarettes have been paired thousands of times in just one year with many activities that you perform everyday. What are some of the activities that for you typically go together with smoking?

Activities paired with smoking:

1 _____

2 _____

3 _____

4 _____

5 _____

Making change happen

Becoming smoke free involves breaking both the chemical and the behavioral addictions. However, trying to overcome both at the same time can cause additional stress, which may decrease the chance of success. Therefore, we aim to weaken the behavioral addiction first, before working on the chemical addiction. So we recommend that you focus on the behavioral addiction first. Then, start on nicotine-replacement therapy and gradually taper down the amount of nicotine that your body receives until you no longer need this chemical "crutch." In the meantime, we will provide you with practical skills to help you to become and remain smoke free.

In combating the behavioral aspect, we look at ways to break the links between activities and cigarette smoking, and also look at ways to break the habitual patterns involved in the act of smoking itself. Some strategies for breaking the behavioral habit of smoking are listed in the next section. It is recommended that you choose at least three of these strategies to try out during the first week. There is a record sheet to monitor the strategies that you tried out each day and to record the number of cigarettes smoked each day. Your participation in change is vital. After all, there is a simple truth – things will stay the same unless you start doing things differently.

To recap, to prepare yourself for the day you become smoke free:

- reduce the amount of nicotine and its effects on the brain
- disrupt the routines and behaviors associated with smoking.

It's time to start doing things differently!

Smoking is a habit. It is something you do without much thinking in the same manner day in and day out. Think of all the occasions when you typically have a cigarette. Now, for each of those occasions when you have had a cigarette, think of exactly what you do when you have a cigarette. Think of where you keep your cigarettes, the matches or lighter that you use, and how you take the cigarette out of the packet. Think of how you hold the cigarette while you light it. Think of how you inhale when you smoke. Think of what you do with your other hand when you smoke. Now, think of the number of times you have done all of these actions in your life – that's a lot of practice for the behaviors to become a habit! So, in order to become smoke free, all the little things that you do when you engage in the act of smoking need to be done differently. This will help you to weaken the behavioral addiction. Remember, change happens when you start doing things differently.

How do you break the habit? By starting to make changes in your normal smoking routine. You can vary virtually all smoking behaviors by following the "When, How, Where" principle. That is, vary *when* you have a cigarette. Always have a cigarette first thing in the morning? Then delay it for a few minutes. Vary *how* you have a cigarette. Always have a cigarette along with your cup of coffee in the morning? Then enjoy the coffee on its own, and if you "must" smoke, do it without your cup of coffee nearby. Vary *where* you do it. Often smoke in your favorite armchair while watching television? Then only smoke outdoors (preferably standing up – don't want to get too comfortable!). Or like to read the newspaper or a book when you smoke? Then read at places where smoking is prohibited (e.g., inside a café, or inside an area in your home that you designated as a smoke-free zone). Do nothing else when you smoke! Aim to change all of your smoking routines, and all of the cues that are associated with your smoking behaviors. A particular obvious type of cue is your ashtrays; most smokers have their home littered with several of them. Remove all ashtrays from your house! Some clients like to collect their ugly cigarette butts in a glass jar, to serve as a visual reminder (i.e., disgusting "cue") of what will not go into their bodies anymore once they are smoke free. You can change many things about the habit of smoking – when you smoke, where you smoke, how many cigarettes you smoke at a particular time, and what else you do when you smoke. Even a small change can alter your smoking routine and hence weaken the habit. For an illustration of how to use the "When, How, Where" principle to make changes to your everyday smoking routines, see the diagram entitled *How to change your smoking routine.*

Also there is a list called *Suggestions on what to do differently before "becoming smoke-free day."* This contains a list of tips that will help you to make those behavioral changes. Aim to adopt at least three or four of the strategies every week. The ***Behavioral changes chart*** can be used to record which of these strategies you used, how often you used them, and how many cigarettes you smoked each week. On the same chart, there are also some extra lines where you can write in other strategies that you might come up with yourself, and that you think would be especially helpful for you personally. Remember, while becoming smoke free is quite a challenge, using these strategies is not. These strategies are simple and require no special skills. If you find yourself after one week not having tried even one or two of those strategies, you may not be ready to become smoke free. Then we can explore with you what it is that stands in your way of becoming a non-smoker, and help you to increase your readiness for change.

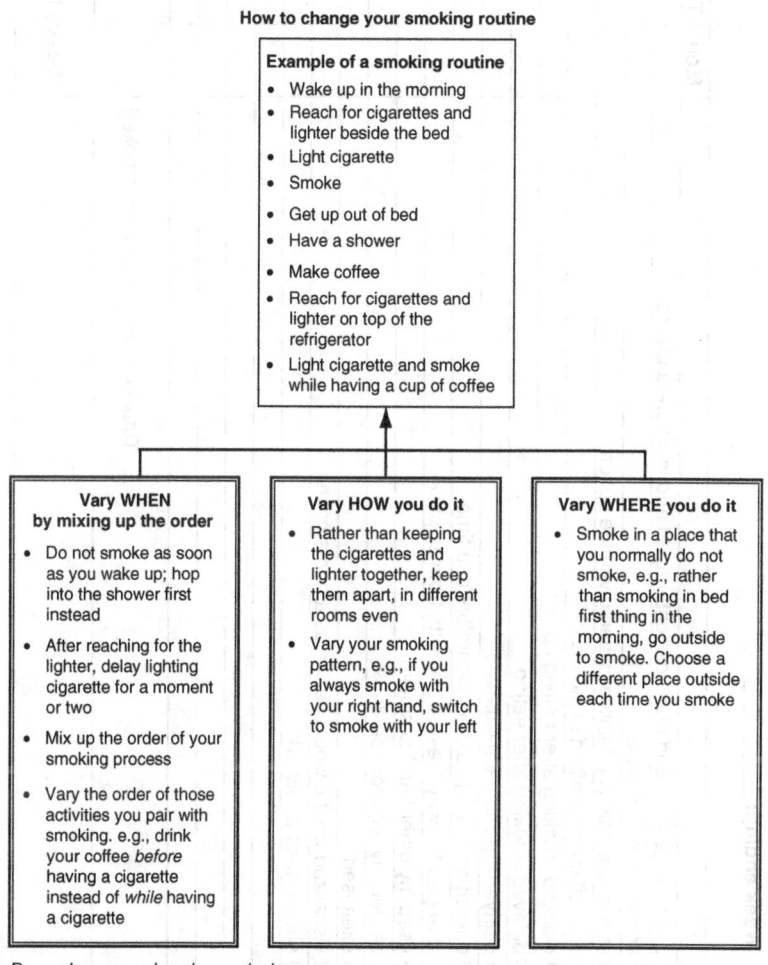

How to change your smoking routine

Example of a smoking routine
- Wake up in the morning
- Reach for cigarettes and lighter beside the bed
- Light cigarette
- Smoke
- Get up out of bed
- Have a shower
- Make coffee
- Reach for cigarettes and lighter on top of the refrigerator
- Light cigarette and smoke while having a cup of coffee

Vary WHEN by mixing up the order
- Do not smoke as soon as you wake up; hop into the shower first instead
- After reaching for the lighter, delay lighting cigarette for a moment or two
- Mix up the order of your smoking process
- Vary the order of those activities you pair with smoking. e.g., drink your coffee *before* having a cigarette instead of *while* having a cigarette

Vary HOW you do it
- Rather than keeping the cigarettes and lighter together, keep them apart, in different rooms even
- Vary your smoking pattern, e.g., if you always smoke with your right hand, switch to smoke with your left

Vary WHERE you do it
- Smoke in a place that you normally do not smoke, e.g., rather than smoking in bed first thing in the morning, go outside to smoke. Choose a different place outside each time you smoke

Remember: vary *when, how* and *where*

Behavioral changes chart

Week ending: _____

	Mon	Tue	Wed	Thur	Fri	Sat	Sun
I put my cigarettes and matches/lighter apart and in different places							
I smoked only outdoors							
I chose non-smoking facilities when given the option							
I did nothing else when I smoked							
I delayed smoking after getting up							
I delayed smoking after eating							
I delayed lighting each cigarette							
I bought only one packet of cigarettes at a time							
I changed the way I take a cigarette from its pack							
I used my other hand to smoke							
I carried my reminder cards							
I exercised							
I visualized what it would be like as a non-smoker							
I gave myself a reward							
Total number of cigarettes smoked							
Weekly total =							

Suggestions on what to do differently before "becoming smoke-free day"

- **Keep a record** of your habit changes and how many cigarettes you smoke each day on your Behavioral changes chart.
- **Stop carrying cigarettes with you.** Put them in a place that is inconvenient and that forces you to make a real effort to get each one (e.g., in the trunk of your car, the hall closet, or the garden shed).
- Stop smoking in your house, in your office, or in your car. **Smoke only outdoors.**
- **Chose non-smoking facilities** when given the option.
- **Do nothing else when you do smoke.**
- After you get up in the morning and after you eat, **make yourself wait** at least 30 minutes before you smoke. Find something else to do instead.
- When you do go to smoke, **hold off for a few moments before lighting up** and think "I don't really need to light this quite yet . . . I can do it in a little while."
- **Get rid of all ashtrays.** You won't need them anymore when you are a non-smoker. Put cigarette butts in an old can or glass; do not empty it, rather keep it to remind yourself what you are putting into your body.
- If you buy cigarettes, **buy only one pack at a time.** Do not "stock up."
- **Change the routine** of how you take a cigarette from its pack (e.g., wrap the pack in paper and put a rubber band around it; this helps to slow down and disrupt the process of lighting up). There are many creative variations to this strategy, select one that will serve as your personalized roadblock and detour to prevent you from lighting up automatically.
- When you do smoke, **use your "other" hand.**
- **Carry some personal reminder cards.** On each card, write down something that you think will encourage you to be a non-smoker. Carry the cards with you where you used to carry your cigarettes. Read them each time you think you are going to have a cigarette.
- Engage in regular **exercise.** Use it to relieve stress and stop urges to smoke.
- Plan your life as a non-smoker. Every day, **visualize** about something that you will do or that will be different once you are smoke free.
- **Give yourself rewards** for doing things differently and following your smoking cessation program.

When to set your "becoming smoke-free day"

We encourage you to think about a day in the next two to four weeks that you want to set as your personal "becoming smoke-free day." Pick a day that you feel gives you a realistic chance to succeed at being smoke free. Prior to that day, you will work hard on the behavior changes. When you are ready, you stop smoking and gradually eliminate the chemical addiction with the help of nicotine-replacement therapy. The difficulty lies not in becoming smoke free (after all, many smokers have "quit" many times in the past, only to resume smoking within hours or days of their quit attempts). Rather, the difficulty lies in remaining smoke free for good. This is why we are less enthusiastic about attempts to quit "cold turkey" right at the start of the program. The scientific evidence suggests that careful planning and preparation for this big moment, or what some have called the "warm turkey" approach, increases the likelihood of long-term success. And it is long-term freedom from smoking we aim for!

- Choose the day you become smoke free carefully.
- Avoid setting a day that coincides with a stressful period or a period of unusually high temptation. Examples of these include the beginning of a stressful working week, or the night of a party where you will be socializing with friends who smoke.
- However, stress and situations where temptations may be present should not be used as an excuse to postpone the day you become smoke free. One is rarely free of all stress or temptation – waiting for a perfect time will keep you stuck in a smoking lifestyle. Instead, choose times when there is relatively less stress. Weekends, holidays, and other special events are good choices.
- Celebrate the day you become smoke free! After all, you're beginning a journey to greater freedom, better health, and a greater sense of accomplishment!
- Mark this day with a ceremony to highlight the significance of the occasion. For instance, flush all remaining cigarettes down the toilet.

On the day you are to become a non-smoker, be sure to get rid of all cigarettes. Do not keep any "for emergencies." If you have a strong urge to smoke, do something else to distract yourself, or use any of the other coping strategies you will learn in this program that will help you to stay smoke free. Remember, if you don't give in to the urge, it will pass soon.

As of this day I stop smoking and start breathing

■	■

From Smoke City to Fresh Hills

Congratulations on deciding to become smoke free! You have decided to embark on a trip to be free from cigarette smoking. As with many journeys, making the move from Smoke City to Fresh Hills is not a case of simply throwing a few things in the car and driving off into the sunset. Rather, journeys take careful planning. This program will provide you with the necessary skills and strategies to make this journey as smooth as possible. Of course, we can only provide you with ways to make the journey smoother – you need to be committed to taking the trip.

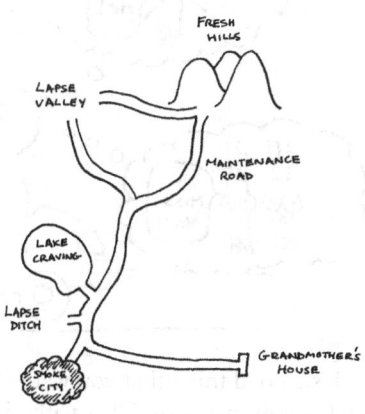

The first thing to do before embarking on your trip is to decide on what to pack and what to leave behind. Things to pack include things that will aid you on the journey. The strategies you learn in this program will be helpful because they will help you cope with any treacherous parts of the journey. You may also want to bring along others who will support you, including the group members. Things to leave behind are those reminders of Smoke City – items such as cigarettes, ashtrays, etc. It may also be wise, at least for a while, to leave behind those Smoke City friends who want to prevent you from making the journey. You can catch up with them when you are firmly settled in Fresh Hills and are able to resist temptations to move back to Smoke City.

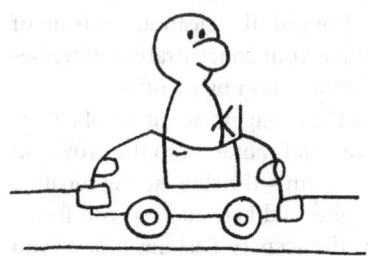

Now that you have packed items that will help rather than hinder you on the trip, you're off! Yes, it might be a teary affair as you leave Smoke City behind, but remember – you're moving on to a better place! So dry those eyes, pull out the map outlining the route from Smoke City to Fresh Hills, and hold on tight for the trip!

Driving along the first leg of your journey, you eagerly look forward to the benefits of living in Fresh Hills and start daydreaming of what life would be like there. One major benefit of living in Fresh Hills is the cheaper cost of living – no cigarette rent collectors. Another benefit is the fresh air up in the mountains. You've been used to breathing in smoke for such a long time. Think of the fresh air filling your lungs with every breath, your improved sense of smell, and even an improved ability to taste. But as you think of the good life that will await you in Fresh Hills, you may wonder if you will make friends there or be able to catch up with your friends living in Smoke City. Then, you start to miss those in Smoke City, and start to reminisce about your days in Smoke City . . . All of a sudden, you snap out of daydreaming and narrowly avoid driving into Lapse Ditch.

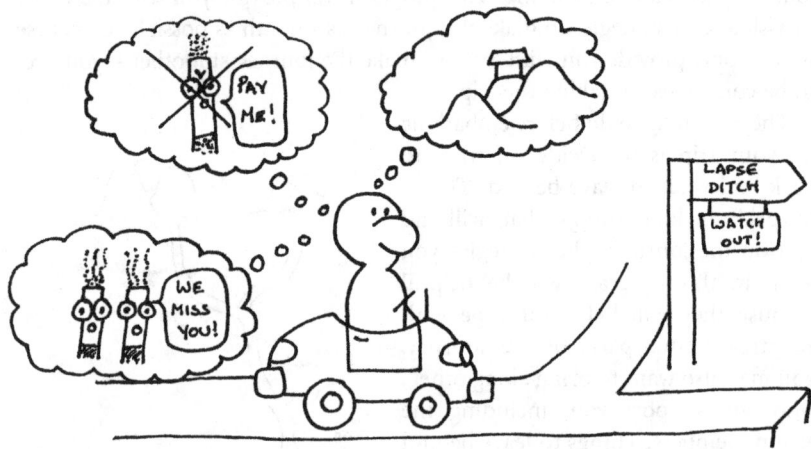

It's a good thing that you were alert just in time! Lapse Ditch is quite deep and certain parts are filled with quicksand that will suck your entire car in. You start to wonder why your mind wandered off. You remember that the journey is a long, unfamiliar one. Moving away from Smoke City and all the fumes and your cigarette friends means that you are not constantly stimulated by nicotine. This may result in feeling tired and bored (from lack of stimulation by nicotine). You may even feel dizzy from all the clean air outside of Smoke City limits. You may also find that at first your concentration decreases somewhat – this also results from a lack of stimulation by nicotine.

Time to take a break now – get free from the thoughts about Smoke City. You pull into the petrol station, fill up your car, and wander into the provision store. There, you decide to buy some nicotine gum – the slow-acting nicotine will take the edge of those Smoke City thoughts and help to keep you fresh.

Back on the road again, and you admire the scenery flashing past as you cruise along. Somehow, things seem very idyllic and peaceful. You notice there's a lake ahead and stop to admire the scenery. Unfortunately, stopping at Lake Craving was a bad idea. It reminds you somewhat of Smoke City and how you and your cigarette friends used to fish by a pond that looked similar to the lake. So you just get back in the car and keep on driving, and Lake Craving eventually passes from your view as you check the rear view mirror, and your thoughts come to focus again on the road ahead.

As you continue on your way to Fresh Hills, you encounter a slippery section on the road. You find it hard to maintain control of your car and it leaves you feeling stressed. You begin to think that you will never make it to Fresh Hills. You also miss your cigarette friends and decide to call them up to meet you in Lapse Valley – a scenic detour on the way to Fresh Hills.

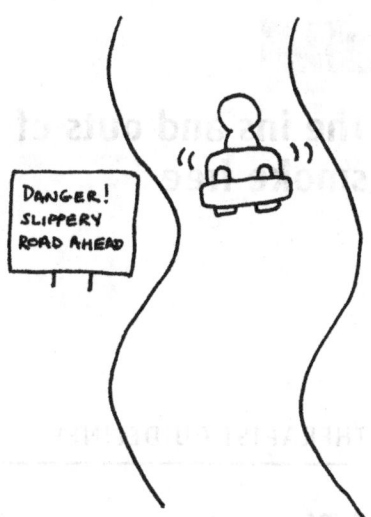

In Lapse Valley, you catch up with your cigarette friends. While they make you feel good initially, you begin to remember why you left Smoke City in the first place. You bid them farewell and continue on your journey.

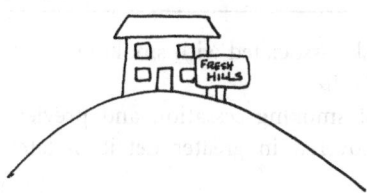

Having left Lapse Valley, you realize you have learnt something about yourself – although you succumbed to the temptation of having a smoke, you realize that you are able to leave it all behind. You learn that although there will be times when you really miss Smoke City, you can move on to your new life in Fresh Hills. You have learnt the skills to do so.

Eventually, you make it to Fresh Hills. You love your new house and the new feeling you have inside. As you sit on the porch, your new neighbor stops by and invites you for a walk to the park. Now that the air is fresher and that you are fitter because you're away from Smoke City, you might just take him up on his offer.

The ins and outs of becoming smoke free

THERAPIST GUIDELINES

Aims

1 Provide information about the health risks associated with smoking
2 Highlight the benefits of becoming smoke free
3 Alert clients to common side effects of smoking cessation and preview some of the coping strategies to be covered in greater detail in later modules
4 Raise awareness about the role of negative moods in smoking behavior and smoking cessation
5 Raise awareness about strategies for coping with mood changes associated with smoking cessation and preview some helpful coping tips to be covered in greater detail in later modules (if applicable)
6 Address concerns about weight gain anticipated from smoking cessation

Health risks associated with smoking

The main points covered in the first segment of this module are: (a) the harmful ingredients contained in a puff from a cigarette, (b) the broad range of health risks associated with smoking, and (c) the health risks of alternative to cigarettes.

What's the harm in a puff?

Your clients probably already know that cigarettes contain highly toxic ingredients, courtesy of advertising campaigns that employ this very strategy in a bid to encourage smokers to quit. Rather than engage in a detailed explanation of each of these ingredients and their toxicity, which may seem more like a sermon from the clients' perspective, encourage clients to glance through the section and highlight anything that they were *not* aware of.

Clients may be surprised by the inclusion of ingredients such as arsenic, 4-amino-biphenyl, lead, and mercury. Two ingredients you should highlight in a bit more detail are nicotine and carbon monoxide (CO).

The addictive nature of nicotine will be known to your clients and has been covered in the first session of the program (Chapter 3). So focus here on its impact on the circulatory and gastrointestinal systems. In particular, highlight the potential damage that nicotine can cause to limbs, particularly in clients who also suffer from diabetes and are, therefore, already susceptible to problems with circulation (specifically, peripheral vascular disease).

Carbon monoxide is another ingredient that is important to highlight to your clients. If carbon monoxide monitoring equipment is available to you, clients would have already received some information about it in their initial assessment session (see client handouts in Chapter 2 entitled *Carbon monoxide (CO) monitoring information sheet* and *Carbon monoxide (CO) feedback chart*). Remind clients in this session that carbon monoxide is found in car exhaust fumes and is what kills people when they try to commit suicide by this method. Important here in the context of general health is to explain the mechanics of the greater affinity that carbon monoxide has for hemoglobin and its impact on oxygen's ability to attach to hemoglobin and how this results in the lack of oxygen to vital cells. A useful analogy presented in the *Client materials* is one of a monorail with limited seats, and clients often find this analogy very helpful.

Review other aspects of health affected by smoking

As with cigarette ingredients, your clients are likely to know many of the health risks associated with smoking. Indeed, some of your clients may have been warned by a concerned partner, doctor, or child that they have to give up smoking because of the health risks to the clients themselves and others around them from exposure to secondary smoke. When discussing these health risks, do so in a matter-of-fact manner and avoid scare mongering, or it may come across as nagging or preaching.

While smokers may be aware of the link between smoking and lung cancer, emphysema, and chronic obstructive pulmonary disease, they often lack knowledge about the link between smoking and poorer general health and mental health (Laaksonen *et al.*, 2006), poorer dental health (Al-Shammari *et al.*, 2006), impaired fertility (Augood, Duckitt, & Templeton, 1998), and peripheral vascular disease (Cole *et al.*, 1993). One straightforward way to introduce these is to ask clients to look over the list of smoking-related health risks in the handout. First, invite comments on any of the information that they are already familiar with, and then on any items in the list that they are not aware of yet.

Here is a good opportunity to personalize this segment of the session. Tailor your discussion to your clients' health concerns gleaned from your initial assessment session to enhance relevance for clients. Generally speaking, it will be much easier to focus on those health risks that are more immediate for the clients; for example, gangrene and the potential need for amputation may not be foremost in the mind of someone who is in their reproductive years and has only been smoking for about five years, but it may be a pressing concern for someone with unmanageable diabetes who has been smoking for many years. Types of health risk that are included in the client handout are: Fertility, peripheral vascular disease, and appearance.

Fertility
There is a link between smoking and impaired female fertility. Typically, this means a longer time to conception, but it is encouraging that fertility returns to normal levels following smoking cessation (Munafò et al., 2002). Smoking also carries with it an increased risk of miscarriage and preterm labor, and it affects neonatal health as CO robs developing cells of the necessary oxygen (Augood et al., 1998). Smoking also has a negative impact on male fertility amongst healthy, fertile men. It affects sperm quality (concentration, motility, and morphology), and is associated with an increased risk of birth defects and childhood cancers in the children (Trummer et al., 2002).

Peripheral vascular disease
Potential limb loss, blindness, heart attacks, and strokes – these are all health risks associated with smoking, and the risks are compounded for clients who have diabetes. While these more extreme effects of smoking are most likely to affect long-term smokers through decades of smoking, these health risks are more immediate if they can be linked with symptoms that clients may already be experiencing. For example, potential limb loss may be linked with existing foot problems such as sores that will not heal, while blindness may attract attention among clients who currently experience some vision loss.

Appearance
Clearly, this is not really a health risk, but it adds to your "bag of tricks" as it is often of more immediate concern to younger clients than cancer, gangrene, and emphysema, which may seem more distant threats. Female clients, in particular, may spend a fortune on antioxidants in a bid to erase facial wrinkles and to look more youthful, and so pointing out that smoking increases facial wrinkling may be helpful. For men, vanity may seem less of a "hook," but highlighting that smoking has been linked with hair loss and

also with impotence (Tengs & Osgood, 2001) can be a way to reinforce their desire to become smoke free.

Discuss the health risks of alternatives to cigarettes

The critical information to convey in this section concerns switching from cigarettes to lower-yield cigarettes, or to alternatives such as cigars. Many clients switch from regular to light cigarettes thinking that these will be less harmful. However, this is often associated with compensatory smoking in order to achieve an equivalent amount of nicotine, even if it is not a conscious decision to do so. Compensatory behaviors include varying puff duration, depth of inhalation, duration of inhalation, number of puffs per cigarette, and the blocking of filter vents (Benowitz *et al.*, 2005; Hammond *et al.*, 2005; Scherer, 1999; see also Box 2.1).

Switching from cigarettes to alternatives because of perceived lower health risks is misguided because many harmful ingredients are common to cigarettes and alternatives. Switching to alternatives is also misguided because of the smoker's established pattern of cigarette smoking. In the instance of someone who switches from cigarettes to cigars, someone who has always smoked cigarettes will inhale more deeply than someone who has only ever smoked cigars, and this same, more intense, pattern of inhalation is likely to be maintained after switching. Moreover, cigar paper is less porous and so smoke is less likely to diffuse into the air, meaning that a cigarette smoker may inhale higher concentrations of smoke from smoking cigars than from smoking cigarettes.

Benefits of becoming smoke free

The main points in the second segment of this module are to (a) highlight that it is never too late to become smoke free and (b) personalize the benefits of becoming smoke free.

It is never too late to become smoke free

Many clients think that there is no point in giving up as they have already done years of damage to their body by smoking and it is too late to turn things around. Indeed, some clients may be in contact with you because they have been referred by their general practitioners but do not believe that becoming smoke free will do *them* much good. The important thing to emphasize with all clients is that *the body starts to repair itself the moment a cigarette is finished,* but it is the continued smoking that impairs this process. Obviously, the earlier one starts this process the better, but even if one becomes smoke free later in life, one can reap many of the significant health benefits described in the client materials (Taylor *et al.*, 2002).

Personalize the benefits of becoming smoke free

Listing the benefits of becoming smoke free will be an incentive for many clients, but personalizing the benefits to the individual client's circumstances makes the message even more powerful in motivating change. A case in point is mortality statistics. Smoking is associated with a shorter lifespan of seven years on average (although there are variations in approximate years gained from stopping at different ages [Taylor *et al.*, 2002]) and a lower number of disease-free years in life relative to non-smokers (Bernhard *et al.*, 2007). Ask your clients to reflect on what that would mean for them in real terms. For example, for a client in her forties, this may mean the difference between seeing or not seeing a child graduate from university or starting off their career. For others, this may mean living long enough to experience the joys of getting to know a grandchild.

Living longer is only one potential benefit of becoming smoke free. As is emphasized throughout this program, living a better quality life is an important and more immediate benefit of becoming smoke free (see also Chapter 10). Anticipated improvements in quality of life from becoming smoke free will, therefore, be an important tool for motivation enhancement, perhaps especially so for younger clients who may feel that mortality statistics are less relevant to them. From your initial assessment of clients' reasons for attending the program, you will have gained an understanding of their motivating factors. These may include appearance (e.g., whiter teeth, not smelling of cigarette smoke), improved finances, less social alienation, and better health. Keep a mental note of your clients' motivations and weave these into the discussion when presenting this module.

Common side effects of smoking cessation

This brief segment is meant to provide clients with a preview of some of the unpleasant temporary changes that they may experience following quit day. Go over the table in the client materials that lists the side effects that are common following the sudden withdrawal of nicotine, along with the reasons why these symptoms occur, and what some of the strategies are to deal with them. The idea is to prime clients as to what to expect and to reassure them that there are a range of effective strategies that will help them to cope with these challenges. Point out to clients that subsequent modules in the program will cover in greater detail strategies on how to manage withdrawal distress and craving and how to prevent and manage a lapse during this difficult period of initial abstinence from nicotine. Emphasizing the suite of strategies available to clients for maintaining abstinence in the face of strong side effects is a helpful step in enhancing self-efficacy.

Negative moods and smoking: awareness and coping strategies

The purpose of this segment is twofold; to take the opportunity early in the program to raise awareness about how negative mood and concerns about weight gain can affect smoking behavior and smoking cessation, and to preview some helpful coping tips. It is useful to raise these issues early in the program as they can constitute barriers to clients' ability to effectively engage in change behaviors and become smoke free. But these issues may not necessarily be of particular concern to every group member. Therapists should, therefore, determine to what extent they are applicable to the members of a given group and then flexibly select the relevant components of later modules to offer tips on handling mood changes and weight concerns during smoking cessation. Of course, the treatment of depression in group members is beyond the scope of the smoking cessation program. The aim here is limited to offering some coaching on how to manage negative moods in everyday situations so that they are less likely to interfere with the goal of becoming smoke free. This is done by using a stepped-care approach. First introduce to clients in this module the *Daily mood log* as a way to assess the extent to which their smoking behavior and change efforts are affected by daily moods. Second, discuss with clients the fact that thoughts and feelings have a strong impact on smoking behaviors and ask clients if they would find it helpful to learn more about these links. If applicable and desired by group members, the module covered in Chapter 9 on *Thoughts: how they affect smoking behavior* can be incorporated in the program in a later session. Finally, provide information on pharmacological options available to smokers with a history of depression and, if appropriate, offer referral options for cognitive–behavioral treatments to those clients who believe that their goal of becoming smoke free could be facilitated with the support of professional help.

Depression and smoking cessation

Smokers are more likely to experience depression symptoms compared with non-smokers, and depressed smokers are less than half as likely to quit than are non-depressed smokers. Smokers are also more likely to experience a depressive episode following cessation of smoking (Anda *et al.*, 1990; Morrell & Cohen, 2006; Wilhelm *et al.*, 2006).

Increasingly, focus has shifted from the impact of depression history on abstinence to the impact of moment-to-moment depressive symptoms or negative affect. It has been demonstrated that current depressive symptoms or recent increased negative affect is predictive of lapse (Kahler *et al.*, 2002), even if smokers do not currently meet a diagnosis of major depression (Berlin & Covey, 2006). Lapses were more likely to occur following the presence of elevated negative affect in the six hours preceding the lapse, and following common everyday stressors, than as a result of more significant but less frequent events (Shiffrin & Waters, 2004). Smoking in this context serves the role of regulating negative affect. Clinically, raising clients' awareness of the potential for "daily hassles" to increase the potential for relapse can have a positive therapeutic impact in itself. Ask clients for examples of this in their lives. For instance, does having a cigarette break feel like a way of obtaining "time out" from a stressful situation. Encourage clients to monitor the link between stressful events, their mood, and the desire to smoke by using the *Daily mood log* in the handout. Box 4.1 contains a description of the log.

Box 4.1. Instructions for using the *Daily mood log*

The aim of the *Daily mood log* is to help clients to recognize patterns in their triggers for stress and depressed mood, and to allow them to monitor situations that can lead to an increased risk for a lapse.

The log is divided into seven rows so that clients can use one sheet for one week.

In the two left-hand columns, clients fill in the date and their overall mood rating for that day. Higher ratings reflect more positive mood.

The third column is for clients to list particularly challenging situations that occurred on that day. In the fourth column, they rate their mood in response to the challenging situation, where higher ratings reflect more positive mood. In the fifth column, clients rate the intensity of their craving in response to the challenging situation, with higher ratings reflecting greater intensity.

Following the introduction of the *Daily mood log*, point out that there is also a link between *unhelpful thoughts* and feelings, and that these feelings can be better managed by turning unhelpful thoughts into more helpful thoughts. Depressed smokers express lower confidence in their ability to refrain from smoking compared with non-depressed smokers. Self-efficacy has been demonstrated to be a predictor of cessation and relapse (Abrams *et al.*, 2000; Norcross, Mrykalo, & Blagys, 2002); it mediates the relationship between depression and abstinence rates (Cinciripini *et al.*, 2003), and individuals with low self-efficacy are less likely to remain abstinent (John *et al.*, 2004;

Morrell & Cohen, 2006). The same unhelpful thoughts that render an individual more vulnerable to depression can also decrease motivation and self-efficacy regarding one's ability to cope without resorting to cigarettes (Berlin & Covey, 2006). For example, unhelpful negative thoughts such as "I don't know why I bother, I'll never be able to quit anyway" can hold clients back from becoming smoke free. If clients show interest in learning more about how thoughts can affect their smoking cessation efforts, tell them that they can learn practical strategies to manage these in subsequent modules (Chapter 9). Modules 3 and 4 on *Kicking the chemical habit* and *Enhancing motivation for change* should be covered first. Module 6 on *Thoughts: how they affect smoking behaviors* could even wait until after Module 5 has been covered on *Prevention and management of a lapse*, unless clients express a particularly urgent interest in learning more about the link between thoughts and feelings sooner in the program. In that case, segments of Module 6 can be introduced along with the material from Modules 3–5.

Finally, it is useful to briefly discuss referral options and pharmacological options available to smokers with a history of depression. Depressed smokers often smoke to self-medicate, as nicotine is linked with increased dopamine and pleasure sensations. The withdrawal of nicotine is, therefore, typically associated with decreased mood. Clients with a history of depression may be particularly interested in bupropion (Zyban), which is an antidepressant that is offered as a pharmacological option for smoking cessation (Chapter 5 has a more detailed discussion). Some research has indicated that while buproprion is beneficial for highly dependent smokers, the depression returns when the bupropion is ceased (Lerman *et al.*, 2004). Similarly, a study of the use of fluoxetine has been shown to enhance abstinence rates when administered together with cognitive–behavioral therapy for smoking; however, abstinence rates are reduced after cessation of pharmacological therapy, presumably as the fluoxetine buffers the mood decrease associated with lower levels of dopamine resulting from smoking cessation (Spring *et al.*, 2007). Clients considering pharmacological treatments for their depression should be advised to consult with their general practitioner.

Weight gain and smoking cessation

The fear of weight gain can be a significant deterrent for clients to become smoke free (Chapman, Wong, & Smith, 1993). While concerns about potential weight gain are more common among women, a significant proportion of men also express concern (Clark *et al.*, 2006), as do older, medically ill smokers (Sepinwall & Borrelli, 2004). The reality is that postcessation weight gain is a concern for many smokers, and this needs to be addressed realistically with clients. Estimates of the amount of weight gain varies, from about

2–4 kg in the first year (Filozof, Fernandez, & Fernandez-Cruz, 2004), to an average weight gain of around 8 kg in a five-year follow-up from the Lung Health Study (O'Hara *et al.*, 1998). It will be important to gauge client expectations regarding weight gain. For example, a survey of women concerned about postcessation weight gain indicates that while they expected to gain approximately 7 kg, they were only willing to tolerate a gain of 2 kg (Levine, Perkins, & Marcus, 2001). Consequently, managing client expectations regarding weight gain, and assisting them to consider the "pros" of continuing to smoke (weight control) in light of the "pros" of becoming smoke free (better overall health and appearance) will be critical in enhancing motivation to become and remain smoke free. The following steps are recommended.

Explain mechanisms of postcessation weight increase. Because nicotine is a stimulant, the body's metabolic rate is higher amongst smokers (Cabanac & Frankham, 2002; Wack & Rodin, 1982). However, the most significant contributing factor to postcessation weight gain is increased caloric intake (Leischow & Stitzer, 1991; Wack & Rodin, 1982). Ask clients to reflect on how smoking stops them from eating; for example, to have a cigarette may mean that they leave the dinner table and are, therefore, less likely to have another helping. Or smoking may be used to help to cope with negative emotions like sadness and boredom in place of emotional eating. The aim here is to help clients to recognize that there is a strong behavioral component to postcessation weight gain, and that they are active agents in managing that behavioral component. Point out that nicotine-replacement therapy can delay postcessation weight gain (Cabanac & Frankham, 2002; Filozof *et al.*, 2004; Jorenby *et al.*, 1996), thus allowing clients to develop alternative behavioral strategies for longer-term weight management.

Emphasize the impact of smoking on appearance. Clients who use smoking to control their weight are also likely to be concerned about their overall appearance. Ask clients what else they do to maintain their appearance – exercise, invest in facials, invest in creams to decrease wrinkles, teeth bleaching, ingesting antioxidants, etc. – and use this to highlight that smoking undermines their attempts to look youthful as cigarette smoking accelerates the aging process (Bernhard *et al.*, 2007). Highlight that smoking is associated with increased facial wrinkling, including the characteristic wrinkling around the mouth of smokers (Koh *et al.*, 2002; Petitjean *et al.*, 2006).

Emphasize the impact of smoking on fat distribution. Explore where weight gain is least tolerated by clients. Discuss with clients that smoking alters the distribution of fat, such that while smokers may have lower overall weight compared with non-smokers, they have a higher waist-to-hip ratio owing to the effects of smoking on the endocrine system, and this effect is reversed when clients quit smoking (Canoy *et al.*, 2005; Jensen *et al.*, 1995; Lissner *et al.*, 1992). Personalize the relevance of this for your clients: for men, a "beer gut" is often viewed as unattractive, whereas for women the ideal is often the hourglass figure and a toned stomach, whereas cigarette smoking promotes an "apple" body shape.

Discuss smoking within the greater context of overall health. In addition to highlighting the impact of smoking on appearance, ask clients to consider what health reasons lie behind their desire to become smoke free. This can mean feeling more fit, feeling healthier, or minimizing the impact of existing damage from smoking. In sum, encourage clients to weigh the cost of a potential modest weight gain against the benefits of vastly improved overall health and appearance.

Introduce an action plan for clients. Having highlighted that clients have a significant impact on postcessation weight gain through increased caloric intake, encourage clients to engage in an action plan for weight maintenance: focusing on regular physical activity, healthy eating patterns, and keeping a check on eating as a substitute for smoking. Suggest making changes straightaway so that they can become established in a new routine before they need to focus their energies on adjusting to a non-smoking lifestyle after their quit day. Above all, encourage clients to maintain their focus on becoming and remaining smoke free, rather than get caught up in focusing on minimizing weight gain.

Tips for working with individuals

This module is introduced in the earlier sessions of the smoking cessation program, and it presents clients with information related to health risks associated with smoking, benefits of becoming smoke free, as well as providing information about common concerns for clients intending to quit, namely depression and weight gain. This module serves as a complement to the motivational chapters (Chapters 6 and 7).

It is very likely that your client has received numerous messages regarding the health risks associated with smoking. It is even possible that some of your clients may be desensitized as a result of some of the scare campaigns run by health departments in a bid to increase quit rates. In order to maintain your client's interest, tailor your discussion of this module to the main health-related concerns presented by the individual client at assessment; the remainder of the information contained in the client materials can serve as a reference for the client if interested. Of course, the same holds when working with a single client rather than with a group. Some examples of how this module may be tailored to individual clients are given below.

Tips (cont.)

A client in her late twenties, planning to start a family, with a history of depression: in working with this individual, you can:
- focus on the impact of smoking on conception and pregnancy
- discuss the impact of low mood on smoking cessation and the benefits of considering a referral for cognitive–behavioral treatment for depression (especially since antidepressant medication may not be a preferred option while pregnant).

A client in his late sixties, with diabetes and coronary heart disease, who has presented on advice of his doctors but feels that there is no point to quitting because of the extensive damage he has already done to his body through decades of smoking. As a compromise, he has switched to light cigarettes. In working with this individual, it may be necessary to:
- dispel myths associated with switching to light cigarettes and discuss compensatory smoking
- discuss the impact of smoking on diabetes and coronary heart disease
- emphasize that there are still health benefits to be gained from becoming smoke free at his age and, importantly, translate this into something tangible for the client: for example, being around to enjoy all the retirement plans he has made with a greater level of fitness.

An executive who feels that smoking is a weakness but smokes in order to cope with stress and to manage her weight. In working with this individual, you can:
- explore what it is about smoking that is a weakness – is it the social stigma associated with it, the dependence on a substance, or a lack of ability to cope with her concerns on her own?
- discuss alternate coping strategies, particularly in the management of stress and weight.

Importantly, maintain your overall focus on helping your client to *become smoke free*. Defer addressing underlying issues to a later date, or consider referral options so that the focus of your sessions remains on becoming smoke free.

CLIENT MATERIALS

1 Health risks associated with smoking
2 Benefits of becoming smoke free
3 Common side effects associated with becoming smoke free
4 Smoking, depression, and weight gain
5 Daily mood log.

Health risks associated with smoking

What's the harm in a puff?

In your journey to becoming and remaining smoke free, you are taking an active step towards cleansing your body of over 4000 chemicals contained in cigarettes, over 40 of which are known carcinogens. Nicotine, carbon monoxide, and tar are just three of these compounds; let's look more closely at what these chemicals do to your body.

Nicotine

Nicotine, a stimulant, is what makes cigarettes addictive. It is associated with an increase in blood pressure and heart rate and an increased likelihood of blood clotting. Nicotine also acts to constrict your blood vessels in your extremities, leading to decreased skin temperature and, in extreme cases, to gangrene. Nicotine use also impacts on the gastrointestinal system, specifically bowel activity (with occasional diarrhea). Finally, because nicotine is so addictive, it keeps you smoking and, therefore, keeps you exposed to all of the other harmful ingredients found in cigarettes.

Carbon monoxide

Carbon monoxide is a colorless, odorless, toxic gas that is found in car exhaust fumes. Carbon monoxide has a devastating effect on the body, robbing living cells of the oxygen that is vital for their functioning. This occurs because carbon monoxide interferes with the ability of oxygen to attach to hemoglobin, which transports the oxygen around the body to our organs where oxygen is needed. It is 200 times easier for carbon monoxide to attach itself to hemoglobin than it is for oxygen to do so.

One way to visualize the impact of carbon monoxide is to imagine a monorail (hemoglobin) that goes around the body. There are only limited seats on the monorail, so the faster the passengers are, the more likely they are to get to the seats. Carbon monoxide is like the faster passengers who can rush in quickly, and the slower passengers – oxygen – are left standing on the platform.

As a result of inhaling carbon monoxide, less oxygen reaches your heart, brain, and lungs, as well other organs. This means that mental and physical functioning slows down, and effects include impaired vision and shortness of breath, as well as decreased mental sharpness.

Tar

Tar is what causes those unsightly stains on smokers' teeth and fingers. Cosmetic implications aside, tar contains several carcinogens. Tar is absorbed by the lungs and harms lung cells, and because smoking also kills off the fine hairs along the upper airways that combat infection, tar can move further down the lungs, causing greater damage.

Other harmful ingredients

Of course, you may already be aware of the effects of nicotine, carbon monoxide, and tar, and these may even be one important reason for you to become smoke free. However, have you considered all of the other ingredients that you ingest every time you have a puff? In the table below are some of the other harmful ingredients found in cigarettes. Keep this list in a prominent place – maybe even inside your box of cigarettes – and look at the list every time you are tempted to light up.

Harmful ingredient	Notes
4-Amino-biphenyl	Known human bladder carcinogen; acute inhalation results in headaches and urinary burning
Acetone	Found in nail polish remover
Acetic acid	Also known as vinegar
Ammonia	Found in toilet cleaner; it is used to enhance the effect of nicotine
Arsenic	A known poison and carcinogen
Benzene	Used in making dyes, synthetic rubber; a known carcinogen
Cadmium	A poisonous metal used to make batteries, a carcinogen
Cyanide	Poison
DDT	Banned insecticide
Ethyl carbamate	Probable carcinogen
Indenopyrene	Carcinogen
Mercury	Heavy metal
Nickel	Carcinogen
Polycyclic aromatic hydrocarbons	Carcinogen

Flavorings

Flavorings are added to cigarettes to enhance their taste. Ingredients listed voluntarily by tobacco companies in Australia, such as British America Tobacco (2006) and Philip Morris Limited (2006), include vanilla extract, raisin juice, apple juice, cocoa, and honey, as well as not so familiar chemicals like hexyl acetate, hexanoic acid, ethyl hexanoate, ethyl acetate, and benzyl cinnamate. The effects of these ingredients when burned – as is the case when you light up a cigarette – are as yet unclear; however they may potentially produce toxic chemical compounds. Cocoa, for instance, produces bromide gas when burnt; this dilates the airways of the lung, thereby increasing the body's ability to absorb nicotine.

What else does smoking do to your health?

You are probably aware that smoking is associated with lung cancer, emphysema, and heart disease, because of the countless advertising campaigns that have warned of these health risks associated with smoking. However, there may be some health risks that you are not aware of.

Smoking causes many types of cancer. That smoking is associated with lung cancer is something that you probably already know. However, smoking is also associated with an increased risk of cancers of the esophagus, stomach, pelvis, stomach, liver, kidney, uterus, pancreas, bladder, kidney, larynx, mouth, and nose.

Smoking affects your respiratory system. Your lungs act as a filter, cleaning to maintain optimal functioning. Cigarette smoke introduces small particles into your lungs, making it difficult for your lungs to cope with additional pollutants. Cigarette smoke damages your respiratory tract and is linked with lung diseases such as bronchitis, emphysema, and pneumonia.

Smoking affects your cardiovascular system. The cardiovascular system includes the heart and circulatory system. Your heart pumps oxygen-rich blood, and your circulation system carries the blood to all parts of your body where it is used by your organs. Nicotine constricts your blood vessels, meaning that oxygen cannot move as effectively around your body as it can in the body of a non-smoker. There is also less oxygen in your body because carbon monoxide has greater affinity for hemoglobin than does oxygen. In all, less oxygen reaches your living cells, and all cells need oxygen to survive. The health effects of smoking include being at increased risk of stroke, hypertension, and having a heart attack.

Smoking affects your eyes. Macular degeneration is a condition characterized by blurred or distorted vision, and is a leading cause of blindness. While macular degeneration mainly affects the elderly, there is increasing evidence to show that smoking accelerates the development of macular degeneration, thus contributing to blindness. Research demonstrates that smokers are two to five times more likely to develop macular degeneration than those who have never smoked.

Smoking affects your hormones. Smoking has a significant impact on your endocrine system. The endocrine system includes the thyroid, pituitary gland, pancreas, ovaries, and testes and is responsible for repairing the body, for growth, digestion, sexual reproduction, and for maintaining internal balance. Smoking modifies fat distribution in the body so that more fat is deposited on the upper body. It decreases the production of estrogen and is linked with early-onset menopause as well as an increased likelihood of an irregular menstrual cycle. Smoking affects insulin and consequently increases your risk of developing diabetes.

Smoking affects your sex life. Smoking can have a significant impact on your sex life as it restricts blood flow to sexual organs. There is evidence linking smoking with impotence. Men who smoke experience difficulties attaining and sustaining erections. Similarly, in women, blood flow to the sexual organs enhances sensation and arousal, and as smoking decreases blood flow, sexual arousal is likely to be diminished.

Smoking affects fertility. Smoking also has a negative effect on fertility. Female smokers who smoke in the year before conception experience delays in the time to conception. Smoking increases the risk of miscarriages, lower infant birth weight, and smoking in pregnancy is associated with an increased risk in the child developing sudden infant death syndrome (SIDS). Maternal smoking in pregnancy is associated with a twofold increased risk for SIDS, and maternal smoking accounts for over 20% of all SIDS. For men, smoking may affect sperm quality (size, shape, and movement); however this area has not been as well researched as the link between smoking and female fertility, and the results are not yet conclusive. Finally, smoking has been linked with early onset of menopause (i.e., one to two years).

Smoking affects your oral health. One obvious effect of smoking on your oral health is that it stains your teeth. However, smoking also increases your risk of gum disease, can delay wound healing, and increases your risk for oral cancer.

Smoking affects your bones. Smoking is linked with a greater rate of bone loss, decreased calcium absorption, as well as an increased risk of falls. By smoking, you increase the lifetime risk of developing vertebral fractures (by 10% in women and by 30% in men) and hip fractures (by 30% in women and by 40% in men). The difference between lifetime risk estimates vary for men and women; this is likely because of the protective effects of estrogen and the greater number of cigarettes smoked by men.

Alternatives to cigarettes also pose health risks

Given the hazards of smoking cigarettes, many smokers often look to alternatives, including "mild" or low-yield cigarettes, cigars, and also herbal cigarettes. The reality is that these alternatives also pose health risks.

Mild or low-yield cigarettes. Smokers often switch to mild cigarettes with the belief that by decreasing the amount of nicotine, carbon monoxide, and tar they decrease the health risks. Low-yield cigarettes differ from regular-yield cigarettes in a variety of ways, including a greater number of perforations in the cigarette filter (to dilute cigarette smoke with air) and the use of more porous paper. The main problem with low-yield cigarettes is that smokers unintentionally change their smoking behaviors when they switch to them. Such compensatory behaviors include increasing the number of cigarettes smoked each day, taking stronger puffs, taking more puffs, taking larger puffs, smoking to a shorter butt length, as well as expelling less smoke from the mouth. Blocking filter vents with fingers or lips to increase the concentration of the hit is also a common behavior.

Cigars. While cigars contain the same toxins and carcinogens as those found in cigarettes, they differ in two significant ways. One difference is that there is a higher acidity level in cigars, which makes the nicotine more accessible and more easily absorbed than in cigarettes. Cigar smokers, therefore, inhale less than do cigarette smokers to get a hit of nicotine. The greatest problem facing smokers who switch from cigarettes to cigars is the smoking behavior. Cigarette smokers "carry over" their habit of inhaling when they switch to cigars. The difficulty with this is linked to the second difference between cigars and cigarettes – cigar binders and wrappers are less porous than cigarette paper, which means that there are higher levels of carbon monoxide in cigar smoke than in cigarette smoke. Consequently, in switching over from cigarettes to cigars, smokers end up inhaling higher concentrations of carbon monoxide than they normally do.

Herbal cigarettes. Smokers often think that because a cigarette is "herbal" it must mean that it is healthier. Some types of herbal cigarette are blended with tobacco, with these brands containing tar and nicotine. Even if herbal cigarettes do not contain nicotine, they are likely to produce tar and carbon monoxide to a level comparable to conventional cigarettes. Some smokers may view using nicotine-free herbal cigarettes as a way of "stepping down" from cigarette use. This is not ideal as it replicates the hand-to-mouth action that they are trying to kick.

Smokeless tobacco. Smokeless tobacco comes in two forms – oral snuff and chewing tobacco. Both contain nicotine and are highly addictive. Health effects associated with smokeless tobacco use include bad breath, gum recession, tooth destruction, and a slower healing rate of cuts and sores in the mouth. There is also evidence to suggest a link between the use of smokeless tobacco and cancers of the mouth and pharynx.

Benefits of becoming smoke free

By becoming smoke free you stand to gain many health benefits. One of the most significant benefits is that you will live longer, regardless of how old you are when you become smoke free. You may think, especially if you have smoked for a long time, that it is too late to change and that the damage has already been done. However, the good news is that your body starts to repair itself the moment you finish a cigarette: within 20 minutes of finishing a cigarette your heart rate decreases, within 12 hours the carbon monoxide levels in your body return to normal, within two weeks to three months your risk of a heart attack begins to decrease, and your risk of coronary heart disease relative to a smoker is halved after just one year. It is by lighting up *again* that smoking is able to continually damage your body. Take a closer look at the longer-term health benefits of becoming smoke free.

- The risk of death relative to continuing smokers decreases almost immediately, and continuous abstinence for at least 10 to 15 years decreases the risk of death to a level comparable to never-smokers.
- The risk of lung cancer decreases, and after 10 years of abstinence it drops below half of the risk for continuing smokers.
- The risks of mouth, throat, and esophageal cancers are halved after five years of abstinence.
- The risk of bladder cancer is halved after a few years of abstinence.
- The risk of coronary heart disease attributable to smoking decreases by half following one year of abstinence, and after 15 years of abstinence the risk is similar to a never-smoker.
- The risk of stroke decreases to the same level as that of a never-smoker within 5 to 15 years of abstinence.
- Pregnant smokers who become and remain smoke free in the first three to four months of pregnancy have infants with birth weights comparable to non-smokers and higher than women who smoke throughout pregnancy.
- Becoming smoke free returns the age at natural menopause to one comparable to never-smokers.

The earlier you stop smoking, the greater the number of years you gain relative to those who continue to smoke – at 35, this translates to living for seven to nine years longer, but even at 65 this translates to living for two to four years longer. What does living a few years longer mean for you? Those extra years may mean that you are able to graduate from university, settle down with your partner, drive your business to success, have a family, see your children/grandchildren finish high school, or witness the birth of your grandchild.

One comment that smokers often raise is that everyone has to die of something at some stage, and they may as well enjoy themselves in the process. The reality is that the health effects of smoking on your heart, lungs, hormones, bones, fertility, eyes, brain, and your increased risk for cancer will all impact on your *quality of life* irrespective of how long you live. Hip fractures, heart problems, gangrene, lung problems, decreased vision, and vascular dementia are hardly enjoyable and can have a significant effect on one's quality of life.

Making changes now is not too late! By becoming smoke free you increase your longevity and you improve your quality of life.

Common side effects associated with becoming smoke free

Your body has become accustomed to the many chemicals in cigarette smoke. Depriving your body of these chemicals, as when you start to become smoke free, will result in physiological changes to your body. Most notably, the effects of going "cold turkey" – that is, without first gradually reducing the number of cigarettes you smoke per day, and without the aid of nicotine replacement – will be most prominent as your body copes with the initial shock of nicotine withdrawal. Using nicotine-replacement therapy can go a long way to alleviating many of these symptoms. The table below lists some side effects that you can expect, as well as steps that you can take to counteract them.

Symptom	Cause	What to do
Tenseness, irritability	Withdrawal from nicotine	Use nicotine patches, engage in relaxation, and exercise
Fatigue	Nicotine is a stimulant	Rest, modify your routine to lighten your workload, and use nicotine patches
Cravings	Withdrawal from nicotine, which is strongly addictive	Nicotine patches, distract, delay, and do something else
Concentration difficulties	Nicotine is a stimulant	Modify your workload and understand that it may take you longer to accomplish tasks
Constipation	Intestinal movement decreases briefly owing to lack of nicotine	Add fiber to your diet and drink plenty of water
Hunger	Cravings may be confused with hunger, and hunger may also reflect a desire for something in the mouth	Drink water or low-calorie drinks, eat low-calorie snacks, or chew gum
Cough, dry throat	Your body is eliminating mucous that previously blocked your airways	Drink lots of water, use cough drops
Sleeping problems	Nicotine affects brain wave function, which influences sleep patterns	Avoid caffeine, use relaxation techniques, and engage in low-stress activities

Some of these symptoms may be difficult to tolerate, but bear in mind that they only last between a few days (for example, coughing or dry throat) and a few weeks (for example, constipation lasts for 1–2 weeks, whereas irritability and fatigue may persist for 2 to 4 weeks). Be kind to your body during this time – try not to subject it to additional stress, and ensure that you make an extra effort to exercise or to relax. Later in the program, when you learn the strategies for preventing and managing a lapse, you will receive more detailed tips on how to manage withdrawal distress and cravings.

Smoking, depression, and weight gain

For some smokers, there are two very significant barriers that stand in the way of becoming smoke free: depression and weight gain.

Depression

It is not surprising to experience a dip in mood when quitting smoking when you consider that nicotine stimulates the "reward" pathway in the brain. When you have been smoking for an extended period of time, your brain will adjust to a heightened level of stimulation in your "reward" pathway, and becoming smoke free results in a decreased level of stimulation through a lack of nicotine.

If you have a history of depression, knowing that a decrease in mood is linked with becoming smoke free can be quite daunting and may even work against your desire to quit. The good news is that research has shown that having a history of depression does not automatically mean that you are doomed to relapse. Rather, it is the moment-to-moment stress that you experience that is more likely to predict a lapse. If you are concerned about mood changes use the *Daily mood log* to help you to chart your daily moods and to identify situations that are particularly stressful for you. This can help you become aware of when negative moods are triggers for your smoking.

Giving up smoking can sometimes feel like a struggle – it is very easy to feel hopeless about your moods, and when you feel hopeless the easiest thing you can think of to help yourself is to reach for a cigarette. The problem is that having a cigarette won't actually solve the problem; it only postpones it for later. This is much like procrastinating on a task – you are still faced with it eventually. Furthermore, the relaxing effects of having a cigarette is only psychological – nicotine is a stimulant and, therefore, does not serve a relaxing function.

Instead, let's look at alternative ways of coping with your moods and with the situation. To do this, we can draw on problem-focused strategies (these address the cause of your stress and low mood) and emotion-focused strategies (dealing with managing the resulting emotion, rather than the source of the problem). Problem-focused strategies are ideal; however, there will be instances where you are not able to modify the source of the problem or when your emotions feel so overwhelming that they need to be addressed, in which case emotion-focused coping strategies are ideal. If this is relevant to you or some of the other group members, we can cover problem-focused coping skills such as time management, problem solving, assertiveness, and goal setting further on in this program. Likewise, we can look later at emotion-focused coping strategies. For example, we can look at how your thoughts about a situation affect the way that you feel. By correcting unhelpful self-talk, your mood can improve, thereby decreasing the need to smoke. At the end of this chapter is a *Daily mood log*, which you can use to help keep track of how your craving for a cigarette is linked to mood.

Exercise is also a powerful technique that you can use to help you to manage low mood. Individuals who exercise following becoming smoke free tend to report stable levels of mood, whereas those who do not exercise after becoming smoke free are more likely to report an increase in negative mood.

Another way to stimulate the reward pathway without resorting to smoking is to incorporate enjoyable activities into your routine. Enjoyable activities may include having a massage, talking to friends, taking a scenic drive, or relaxing on the beach. Make these a priority – you need to actively incorporate different rewards now that you won't be able to rely on the quick-and-ready "reward" from your regular nicotine fix.

Finally, if you find it difficult to apply any of these strategies in managing possible mood changes while you adjust to a smoke-free lifestyle, or you feel that they are not working as well as they could, consider talking to a mental health professional.

Smoking and your weight

Concerns about weight gain remain a significant obstacle for some people wanting to become smoke free. Approximately half of women and a quarter of men enrolled in smoking cessation treatment express concern about weight gain as a result of no longer smoking. Being too concerned about weight can affect your ability to become a non-smoker.

What to expect

Some weight gain can occur following smoking cessation. Some studies suggest a weight gain of approximately two to four kilograms in the first year, while a five-year follow-up from the Lung Health Study carried out in North America found an average weight gain of around eight kilograms over a five-year period. While it is easy to reach the conclusion that giving up smoking automatically leads to weight gain, let's look in more detail about what factors contribute to weight gain following smoking cessation.

Change in your metabolism. Our bodies have a natural range within which our bodies are programmed to weigh – known as the set point. Nicotine is a stimulant, and it increases the energy that our body uses, which, in turn, lowers the body's set point. Nicotine-replacement therapy has been shown to delay weight gain following smoking cessation; however, it is important to bear in mind that it can only *delay* rather than eliminate weight gain.

Increased energy intake. The effects of withdrawing nicotine on the body's set point is not the only explanation for weight gain following smoking cessation. We also need to look at how smoking behaviors contribute to maintaining lower weight for smokers. Such scenarios may include smokers leaving the dinner table to have a cigarette after a meal, thereby limiting access to extra helpings, or smokers using smoking to cope with negative moods where others may use eating. Possibly the taste of cigarettes may also act as an appetite suppressant for some. Indeed, studies suggest that it is this increase in the calories consumed that is the main cause of weight gain following smoking cessation.

The sensible approach to avoid gaining weight after smoking cessation

While it may be tempting to control your weight by restricting what you eat, dieting can actually hinder your attempt to remain smoke free. Remember, becoming smoke free can be a stressful event, and any further increases in stress levels, such as from dieting, will increase the likelihood of a lapse. Furthermore, by restricting what you eat, you may feel deprived of something that you desire and the danger is that cigarettes suddenly become even more appealing, which, in turn, increases the likelihood of a lapse. To avoid putting yourself in this high-risk situation, adopt a sensible approach to weight management by maintaining a balanced diet and some level of regular physical activity.

The amount of weight that you may gain following smoking cessation is modified by factors such as genetics, level of physical activity, age, and alcohol consumption. Obviously, some of these factors cannot be altered (genetics, age) but the others can be addressed. Overall, it is best to engage in regular physical activity and healthy eating habits. If you think your physicial activity level and eating habits could be improved, you should start making these changes as soon as possible, preferably *before* you become smoke free. The reason for this is that becoming smoke free can be stressful, and having already established some routine of a healthier lifestyle will make the process less stressful.

Exercise

Physical activity is a healthy way to offset any weight gain and to boost your metabolism. It also increases your energy levels, clears your mind, relieves stress, and helps to alleviate depressed mood that you may experience as a result of becoming smoke free. While there are many health benefits of exercising, it can sometimes feel like a chore. To help you get going, keep the following points in mind.

- Start slowly and gradually, and set realistic goals for fitness. If the most that you have previously done is drive to buy your groceries, it will be some time before you can complete a sustained power walk or even a run around the block.
- Try to do at least 30 minutes of some physical activity a day.

- Find an activity that you like, matching it to your stamina and lifestyle. By selecting something that you find pleasurable, exercise becomes something to look forward to.
- Exercise with others – you will feel more accountable and, therefore, be more likely to stick with it.
- Schedule in exercise rather than saving it for when you can squeeze it in. This will avoid exercise being pushed down the list of activities to complete.
- Exercise even when you don't feel like it, especially if it is at the end of a stressful day at work. Tiredness experienced in this situation is likely to reflect mental, rather than physical, strain.
- Reward yourself (with something other than food or a cigarette) for sticking to your exercise routine.
- Finally, make physical activity a lifestyle change that fits into your daily routine. This is the best way to ensure its sustainability. Create opportunities for exercise on a daily basis. For example, if you normally catch the bus to work, get off one stop earlier so that you walk a bit further. Go for a walk during your lunch break. Take the stairs rather than the elevator, or get off the elevator two floors before your floor and take the stairs. Make small changes that get you moving.

Watch what you eat

In the process of becoming smoke free, you may feel at a loss as to what to do with your hands now that you no longer have the hand-to-mouth action of smoking a cigarette. Unfortunately, one substitute for cigarettes that many smokers resort to is food. Instead, aim for a well-balanced diet where you obtain your nutrients from a variety of sources: fruit and vegetables, protein, grains, low-fat dairy, and small amounts of fats, oils, and sugar.

Having a healthy diet does not mean a sentence of celery sticks and cottage cheese if you do not like them. This is an opportunity for you to seek out more creative options. You can also look for healthier alternatives to what you usually eat. Consider baked pretzels rather than chips, salsa rather than a creamy dip, low-fat milk rather than the full-cream variety, grilled foods rather than fried ones, salad as a side rather than chips – there are many ways in which you can make simple modifications.

There may be certain situations that will make you more likely to eat as a substitute for smoking. Be wary of these situations, such as the following examples.

Extra helpings. It is tempting to eat more if you are staying seated at the table because you no longer need to leave to have a cigarette. In this case, try to maximize feeling full – do not do anything else while eating, chew each mouthful slowly, and drink water. Resist second helpings. Select healthy options when they are presented.

Nibbling as a substitute for smoking. Carry gum and lollies as substitutes for high-fat foods, or look for low-fat snacks. Choose foods that require effort to eat, like unshelled nuts and unpeeled fruit (rather than dried fruit). This way, both your hands and mouth are occupied.

Social situations or activities that are typically associated with smoking. These situations are a minefield as eating is often used to compensate for not smoking. Where possible, try to avoid these situations early on in your journey to becoming smoke free so that temptation is minimized. Where unavoidable, hold these activities in places where you will not be tempted by easily available snack foods (e.g., far away from where the snacks are displayed). Finally, watch out for situations where you may consume additional alcohol in place of smoking as it will increase your kilojoule intake; try to alternate your drinks with water if this is the case.

Smoking, weight gain, and appearance: looking at the bigger picture

The prospect of gaining weight can undermine the motivation for becoming and remaining smoke free. One can easily fall into the trap of thinking that a few extra kilograms would have a disastrous impact on one's appearance. In reality, smoking itself damages one's appearance in a number of ways.

Body shape. Smoking can affect body shape in that more fat is deposited around the stomach, thereby increasing the risk of cardiovascular disease. This is because smoking affects hormones that regulate fat distribution. In a large survey of over 20 000 British men and women, current smokers had a higher waist-to-hip ratio than non-smokers, with the number of cigarettes smoked linked with higher waist-to-hip ratios even after accounting for alcohol intake, energy intake, physical activity, and age. Similarly, a Swedish study found that, for women with similar body mass indices, smokers had significantly more upper body fat than non-smokers. If weight is a concern that affects your motivation to become smoke free, it may be helpful to consider whether an increased waist-to-hip ratio is something that you desire – while you may weigh a bit less, you are more likely to develop an apple shape, love handles, or a "muffin top," compared with non-smokers.

Aging. Smoking makes you look older! It is the second biggest cause of premature aging after the sun. Smoking decreases collagen production and reduces oxygen flow to the skin, thereby prematurely aging skin by 10–20 years. Compared with non-smokers and past smokers, current smokers have more wrinkles (in particular around the mouth owing to the action of puffing on a cigarette) and have skin that is more sallow in appearance. Why spend all that money on face creams with antioxidants and on facials to make your skin look brighter when you destroy it by smoking?

Stains and smells. Smoking stains your teeth and your fingers, and you end up smelling of cigarette smoke. Why spend your money on whitening your teeth, on manicures, and expensive aftershave and perfume, only to undo these each time you light up?

The reality is that becoming smoke free has many benefits for both your health and your appearance. What would it mean to you to look younger and not to smell of smoke? What would it also mean for you to be fitter and healthier? While some weight gain may be part of becoming smoke free, you have the ability to take active steps to manage your weight. The many benefits of not smoking clearly outweigh any modest weight gain you may or may not experience.

Daily mood log

How to use the log

The first two columns are for you to rate your daily mood. Fill in the date in the first column. The second column is for you to rate your overall mood for that day from 1 to 10. Higher ratings indicate a more positive mood.

The last three columns are for you to record situations that you experienced that day that were particularly challenging for your mood and your desire to be smoke free. Fill in the situation in the third column. In the fourth column, rate your mood in response to the situation, with higher ratings reflecting more positive mood. In the fifth column, rate how intense your craving was in response to that situation, with higher ratings indicating more intense cravings.

Daily ratings		Particularly challenging situations		
Date	Daily mood rating (1–10)	Specific negative situations	Mood (1–10)	Intensity of craving (1–10)

An example of the Daily mood log

The example log shows how daily stresses affect mood and the craving for a cigarette.

Daily ratings		Particularly challenging situations		
Date	Daily mood rating (1–10)	Specific negative situations	Mood (1–10)	Intensity of craving (1–10)
15/01	5	Found out that I was the only one not invited out to lunch with my friends.	3	4
16/01	8			
17/01	2	Performance review at work.	1	9
		Got home late, argued with my partner.	2	6
18/01	3	Looked through my finances only to realize that I am in more debt than I thought.	1	8
		My brother cancelled plans to catch up.	3	2
19/01	7	Running late for an important meeting.	5	9
20/01	6	Argument with my sister.	4	7
21/01	5	My children were sick so I had to cancel my social plans.	4	4

5

Kicking the chemical habit

THERAPIST GUIDELINES

Aims

1 Review the rationale for using pharmacological aids in smoking cessation interventions.
2 Provide information about nicotine-replacement therapy and bupropion (Zyban).
3 Provide information on how to use "quitting" products correctly and what to consider when choosing between different available products.
4 Provide information on the risks and benefits of combining different pharmacological aids.
5 Review the guidelines with respect to smoking while using pharmacological aids.
6 Emphasize that the evidence for the effectiveness of pharmacological aids is typically based on trials that included some form of additional non-pharmacological treatment or support.

This module on pharmacological aids to smoking cessation is typically introduced in the third group session (i.e., after *Starting the change process* and *The ins and outs of becoming smoke free*). Sometimes it works better to wait until the fourth session (i.e., around the period that group members are encouraged to schedule their quit day) if progress monitoring of the first couple of sessions suggests that engagement in active change behaviors by some group members is still inconsistent. Under those circumstances, it is better to bring forward the module on *Enhancing motivation for change* and apply the motivational interviewing strategies covered in that module first. That is, nicotine-replacement therapy (NRT) and bupropion (Zyban) are normally only used as part of an abstinent–contingent treatment, where smokers must commit to not smoking anymore after their target quit date.

If that commitment is not sufficiently strong, examining and enhancing the motivation for change can increase the chances that smokers will be ready to refrain from smoking while using pharmacotherapy.

The rationale for using pharmacotherapy

When introducing the topic of pharmacological treatments, remind the group members of the two components of nicotine dependence: behavioral and chemical. Both make it hard for smokers to quit, and it would, therefore, be a false hope that taking NRT products or pills alone can make the nicotine addiction go away without also the effort to change behavior. Behavioral and pharmacological approaches compliment each other. The addition of pharmacotherapy to interventions providing support or counseling roughly doubles the odds of becoming smoke free (Hughes, Stead, & Lancaster, 2007; Silagy *et al.*, 2004). Individuals with high levels of nicotine dependence are most likely to benefit from using NRT (Silagy *et al.*, 2004).

The complementary nature of combining behavioral and pharmacological approaches underlies the sequencing of modules in this program. Remind the group members that by engaging in the change behaviors introduced in the first session, they gradually reduced the number of cigarettes they smoked per day (i.e., the "warm turkey" approach). This offers two benefits. First, it places the emphasis on the clients directly implementing change in their smoking behavior and thus does not feed into the false hope that NRT can do all the work for them. Second, as their bodies become used to receiving lower levels of their daily nicotine fix, the gap between the amount of nicotine the brain "wants" and the amount NRT can deliver (which is much less than the amount delivered by cigarettes) has narrowed. This can help to motivate some heavy smokers to try NRT again, even though they report that NRT did not work for them in the past, failing to reduce withdrawal discomfort sufficiently for them. In this way, NRT will build on the nicotine reduction already achieved by behavioral change strategies and continue this gradual weaning off the chemical habit after the nicotine supply from cigarettes is cut off entirely on the day the client stops smoking altogether. The addition of pharmacotherapy can take the edge off any withdrawal distress during this transition period of adjusting to life without nicotine.

Pharmacological treatments and chosing which to use

The client materials provide information on each of the available pharmacological treatments. All forms of NRT and the antidepressant bupropion are equally effective and approximately double the odds of quitting (Hughes *et al.*, 2007; Silagy *et al.*, 2004). The choice between alternative cessation products from this menu of options is, therefore, primarily based on patient preferences, ease of use, costs, and consideration of potential side effects and risks. Group members should be advised to consult with their doctor or pharmacist before using pharmacological treatments. The one non-nicotine product licensed for use in smoking cessation (bupropion) is available only on prescription. Compared with NRT, some of the contraindications and side effects associated with bupropion, which are listed in the client materials, are considerably more serious (Goldstein, 2003). Notably the increased risk of seizures, although rare, is a serious safety concern. There have also been reports of some suicides and deaths while taking bupropion (e.g., Bergmann *et al.*, 2002), but there is insufficient evidence to link these deaths causally to the use of bupropion (Hughes *et al.*, 2007). Given the more benign safety profile of NRT and equal effectiveness across the various products, there is little reason to recommend bupropion as a first choice among pharmacotherapies.

The risks and benefits of combining different pharmacological aids

There is no strong evidence that combining different NRT, or NRT with bupropion, achieves better outcomes than using a single product (National Institute for Clinical Excellence, 2002; Silagy *et al.*, 2004). Some evidence suggests that using a form of ad lib dosing (e.g., gum or lozenges) while using patches can be beneficial in coping with acute urges to smoke (Silagy *et al.*, 2004). Some experts believe that the regulations for NRTs that ensure safety and quality standards are overly restrictive and that warning labels that accompany these products may give a false sense of risk to smokers, compared with the far greater risk of continued smoking (Kozlowski *et al.*, 2007). However, until there is better evidence that combining NRTs, or increased dosing (e.g., using more than one patch at a time), yields better outcomes without increasing side effects and risks, clients should heed the warning labels in the manufacturers' product information and the advice of their healthcare provider.

Guidelines on smoking while using pharmacological aids

Because smoking while using NRT products raises nicotine levels beyond the clients' baseline levels prior to treatment, which may lead to nicotine toxicity, NRT is generally only commenced after quit day. In the special case where baseline levels have first been reduced by at least 50%, the *Cut down then stop* (CDTS) approach as described in the *Client materials* has been approved in 20 countries for nicotine gum and inhaler (ASH, 2007). The manufacturer of bupropion recommends that (a) smokers are fully committed to quitting smoking before starting to take it, (b) continue smoking only during the first week as bupropion reaches its therapeutic level, and (c) stop smoking within the second week of taking the drug (GlaxoSmithKline, 2005). It is noteworthy that NRT products are used by some smokers for the purpose of temporarily abstaining from smoking in situations where smoking is prohibited, rather than as an aid to smoking cessation (Kozlowski *et al.*, 2007). While this is good news for the manufacturers of these products, it may decrease the motivation of smokers to quit in the long term, and hence the net benefit of these products for public health may be diminished.

Pharmacological aids as one of an array of effective strategies

Most experts agree that pharmacological aids can help people to become smoke free, but only if the person wanting to quit is "also willing to put some work into it" (Kozlowski *et al.*, 2007, p. 2145). These products will not make the task easy, but can make it *easier*. Not everyone will find them equally helpful. Keep in mind that, especially for people coming to smoking cessation groups, quitting has not been easy in the past. Most have tried quitting before and even with the use of pharmacological aids were unsuccessful. That is why they seek more intense help now. One should also be mindful of the implicit claims conveyed by typical television commercials that suggest, for example, that NRT products such as gum and lozenges can be used effectively when the urge to smoke hits during a party situation. Because such situations typically involve the consumption of beverages, these oral NRT products will not be that helpful, as drinking beverages right before or during their use interferes with their effectiveness. In sum, while many smokers can benefit from using pharmacological aids as an effective adjunct to making significant changes to their behavior and lifestyle, any false hopes for an "easy fix" should be countered by offering realistic expectations, coaching the correct use of these products to maximize their effectiveness, and integrating their use within a range of effective cessation strategies as part of a committed behavior change plan.

Tips for working with individuals

The module on kicking the chemical habit can be directly applied when working with individual clients. No adaptations of materials or procedures are needed when using this module with an individual client instead of a group. Of course, if an individual client's level of dependence is very low, and/or the client does not experience any significant withdrawal distress, or is already smoking at a light level (i.e., around five or less cigarettes a day), there may not be any need to discuss details of pharmacological aids. In that case, this module can be omitted from the individual treatment plan. This is different from group interventions. Although there is typically at least one client in most groups who fits the profile of a very light smoker with no signs of physical dependence on nicotine or withdrawal distress, most group members would benefit from a combined behavioral–pharmacological intervention, and hence this module is an integral part of group interventions.

For the individuals who at the start of treatment are very light smokers and who can easily go without a cigarette for many hours or even days, it is not uncommon that we find them clinging to just one or two cigarettes a day, while at the same time the "hard-core" smokers have made huge gains in reducing their daily cigarette intake and then gone smoke free with the help of pharmacological aids. For those "clinging" individuals, the one or two remaining cigarettes a day have nothing to do with chemical dependence; they serve a psychological need (e.g., they may be perceived as "friends" to cope with loneliness). In these cases, the strategies discussed in the motivational interviewing and problem-solving modules of this program are more relevant than strategies for quitting the chemical habit.

CLIENT MATERIALS

1 Kicking the chemical habit and use of medications

Kicking the chemical habit and use of medications

The process of becoming smoke free means beating both the behavioral and the chemical habits. Several medications are available that can help with kicking the chemical habit. These medications approximately double the odds of becoming smoke free. It would be wrong to believe, though, that medications offer an easy "medical cure" for the far more difficult problem of beating addictive smoking behavior. In order for you to become smoke free, you need to change your lifestyle and *do things differently*. Pharmacological aids help to take the edge off withdrawal symptoms and can reduce cravings while you engage in the strategies that deal with the behavioral and learned components of nicotine dependence.

You have a choice from among a range of "quitting" products. They are all equally effective and generally safe to use, but they differ in the side effects you may experience and the potential risk associated with their use in some people. Some of these products are also easier to use than others to achieve the maximum benefit from their use.

It is important to discuss your options with your doctor or pharmacist. Use of these products may require careful consideration for people with certain health conditions, for pregnant and breastfeeding women, or for people under the age of 18.

There are two types of pharmacological aid to becoming smoke free: **nicotine-replacement therapy** (**NRT**) and **bupropion** (also known by the trade name Zyban), which is an antidepressant medication that was found also to help people stop smoking.

Nicotine-replacement therapy

Replacement therapy provides the smoker with a smaller, safer amount of nicotine than cigarettes do, without the other harmful parts of cigarette smoke such as tar and carbon monoxide. It does so more slowly than cigarettes, and thus without the rapid nicotine spikes in the brain that follow the inhalation of nicotine from cigarette smoke. This "smoothing" of the rapid nicotine spikes in the brain while controlling the physiological "need" for the drug helps to reduce urges to smoke. It is recommended that all products be used for 8–12 weeks. Should you need to take it for longer, consult with your doctor or pharmacist. People with certain health conditions should also seek the advice of a healthcare professional before using NRT (e.g., smokers with unstable heart disease or acute heart-related problems such as a recent heart attack or stroke, or people undergoing treatment for cancer). Pregnant and breastfeeding women should try to become smoke free without the use of NRT.

Nicotine patch

The nicotine patch works by slowly releasing a constant dose of nicotine, which gets absorbed through the skin. Patches are available in different sizes and deliver between 5 mg and 22 mg of nicotine. They are designed to be worn either for 24 hours or 16 hours. Both types are equally effective. The 16-hour patch is removed before going to bed so that no nicotine is absorbed overnight. For more-dependent smokers and those experiencing strong withdrawal distress upon waking, the 24-hour patch may be more suitable.

How do I use it? Once you have stopped smoking, use one patch per day, gradually decreasing the patch strength over the course of treatment. Apply the patch to a dry, relatively hairless part of your skin. Place a new patch on a different location to avoid irritation.

What do I need to consider? Patches are very easy to use and need only one application per day. In other words, once they are in place, you can forget about them and go on with your daily routine. Patches may cause skin irritations, which typically are mild and can be minimized by moving the location of the patch on your body around from day to day. Avoid patches if you have a skin disorder. The 24-hour patch may disturb sleep or cause vivid dreams. You should not smoke while wearing a patch as this can lead to nicotine toxicity. Because patches release nicotine at a slow, constant rate, they cannot be used for "on the spot" coping with a specific, acute episode of craving.

Nicotine gum

Chewing and holding the gum in your mouth releases the nicotine, which is absorbed through the lining of the inside of your cheeks and lips. Nicotine gum comes in 2 mg and 4 mg strengths. More-dependent smokers should use the higher-strength gum.

How do I use it? To achieve the maximum clinical benefit, a specific technique to chewing the gum must be followed. Compared with patches, the correct use of nicotine gum is initially a bit more difficult because first you have to "unlearn" the way you are used to chewing regular gum. If you chewed it like regular gum then much of the nicotine would simply be swallowed and wasted. Nicotine gum should be chewed *slowly* to release the nicotine and then rested for one minute under the tongue or be "parked" between the cheek and the gums of your teeth. This chew–park–chew technique should be repeated for about 30 minutes. Up to 15 pieces can be used per day at a rate of one piece an hour. Do not drink anything (including citrus juices, coffee, tea, beer, wine, or sodas) for at least 15 minutes before and nothing while using nicotine gum, because this interferes with the nicotine getting absorbed through the lining of your mouth.

What do I need to consider? Unless the gum is used precisely as instructed, nicotine released from the gum cannot be absorbed through the lining of the mouth, and hence there would be little clinical benefit. Side effects may include burning sensation in the mouth, hiccups, mouth ulcers, indigestion, and nausea. Nicotine gum is not suitable for people with dentures. Unlike patches, gum acts faster and hence can provide relief also from sudden urges. Chewing gum may not be acceptable in some professional settings.

Nicotine lozenge

Sucking on the lozenge allows nicotine to be absorbed through the lining of the mouth. Lozenges come in 2 mg and 4 mg (also 1 mg in the UK) strengths. More-dependent smokers should use the higher-strength lozenge.

How do I use it? Allow the lozenge to dissolve slowly in the mouth moving it around from time to time. This may take 20–30 minutes. If not dissolved completely after 30 minutes, it can be removed. Lozenges can be used regularly at the rate of approximately one per hour up to 15 lozenges a day. The number of lozenges used per day should be reduced over the treatment period. Do not drink anything (including citrus juices, coffee, tea, beer, wine, or sodas) for at least 15 minutes before and nothing while using nicotine lozenges, so your mouth can absorb the nicotine.

What do I need to consider? Lozenges are a palatable and discrete method of nicotine delivery. Side effects may include mouth irritation, hiccups, sore throat, nausea, headache, insomnia, flatulence, and indigestion.

Sublingual nicotine tablet

These small 2 mg tablets are placed under the tongue, where they dissolve and release nicotine to be absorbed through the lining of the mouth.

How do I use it? The tablet should be placed under the tongue and allowed to dissolve. It should not be sucked, chewed, or swallowed. If not dissolved completely after 20 minutes, it can be removed. The number of tablets used per day should be reduced over the treatment period. Do not drink anything (including citrus juices, coffee, tea, beer, wine, or sodas) for at least 15 minutes before and nothing while using the tablets, so your mouth can absorb the nicotine.

What do I need to consider? Sublingual tablets are easy to use and they are discrete. They can be used whenever there is an urge to smoke. Taste may initially be unpleasant. Side effects may include local irritation in mouth or throat.

Nicotine inhaler

The inhaler is a small plastic tube loaded with a replaceable nicotine cartridge, which is inserted into a mouthpiece. On inhalation, nicotine vapor is not inhaled into the lungs but is absorbed through the lining of the mouth when air is drawn through it. Each cartridge contains 4 mg of nicotine.

How do I use it? The cartridge is placed inside the inhaler and pierced. "Puff" on the mouthpiece for about 20 minutes. The time each cartridge will last depends on the intensity and number of puffs. The cartridge is replaced after about three puffing sessions or when there is no taste to the vapor. You can use the inhaler whenever you feel an urge to smoke.

What do I need to consider? The inhaler keeps your hands busy and involves puffing, which some smokers find helpful when dealing with urges. On the downside, the hand-to-mouth and inhaling action mimics the same behavior that you do when smoking a cigarette. This will make it more difficult for some smokers to break the strong links between their routine behaviors and smoking and for some this will also make it harder to wean themselves off using the inhaler. Some also find it inconvenient having to carry the inhaler and using it in public or social situations. It takes about 20 minutes of puffing to achieve the maximum benefit. It is, therefore, not that useful when quick relief from an urge to smoke is desired. Side effects tend to be mild and include coughing and throat irritation. In cold weather, inhalers may not be effective unless they can be kept warm at an ambient temperature above 10 degrees Celsius (50 degrees Fahrenheit).

Bupropion (Zyban)

Bupropion is a non-nicotine aid to help smoking cessation. It was originally developed as an antidepressant medication. The exact way in which bupropion helps to abstain from smoking is not known. It is thought that it affects the same pathways in the brain as nicotine does. Bupropion comes in 150 mg tablets and it requires a prescription from a doctor. The manufacturer recommends that you should be fully committed to quitting smoking before you start taking the tablets. Bupropion should be used together with non-pharmacological cessation strategies and support.

How do I use it? Bupropion is a medicine and must only be used as instructed by a doctor. The tablets need to be swallowed whole. Do not chew, divide, or crush the tablets. The usual recommended dose is one tablet a day for the first three days increasing on the fourth day to one 150 mg tablet twice a day. Doses should be taken at least eight hours apart, and the treatment should continue for 7 to 12 weeks. If using bupropion, start about one week before you stop smoking, as it will take about this long for bupropion to reach the right levels in your body to be effective. Within two weeks of starting to take the tablets, you must stop smoking.

What do I need to consider? All medicines have risks and bupropion is not suitable for some people. It is contraindicated for people under 18 years of age and for people who have certain medical conditions, including allergic reactions to bupropion, seizure disorders, head trauma or brain tumor, eating disorders, liver or kidney disorders, concurrent use of medicines called monoamine oxidase inhibitors (MAOIs), or bipolar disorder. It also is contraindicated during pregnancy and while breastfeeding, heavy drinking, or undergoing abrupt withdrawal from alcohol. There are also several medications and even herbal preparations that can interact with bupropion to increase the risk of adverse reactions (e.g., lowering the threshold for experiencing a seizure). It is, therefore, vital to seek the advice from a doctor when considering whether or not taking bupropion is appropriate for you. Like all medicines, bupropion tablets can cause side effects. While most are likely to be minor and temporary, some can be serious. There is a chance that 1 out of every 1000 people taking bupropion will have a seizure. The chance of this happening can increase if any of the above risk factors are present. The most common side effects include headache, difficulty sleeping, upset stomach, dry mouth, and dizziness. The risk factors and possible side effects mentioned so far are not a complete list. Others may occur in some people, and there may be some side effects that are not yet known.

Are there benefits or risks of combining pharmacological aids?

There is not much evidence that combining NRT products is better than using one product alone, although there may be a small benefit from combining the nicotine patch with a product that can provide fast relief from acute cravings, such as gum. Some manufacturers are now offering a combination pack that contains patches and gum. The manufacturer of bupropion cautions that combining NRT with bupropion may raise your blood pressure, and it is best to seek medical advice when considering combining these. If you feel that NRT is not working for you at the recommended dose, do not increase the dose (such as using more than one nicotine patch at a time) without first consulting with your doctor.

Is it "OK" to smoke while taking nicotine replacement or bupropion?

Smoking while using NRT products amounts to "topping up" the level of nicotine in your body, which may lead to nicotine toxicity. Therefore, NRT products should generally be used only *after* quit day. In the special case where a smoker cuts down to 50% of his or her usual level of smoking, nicotine gum

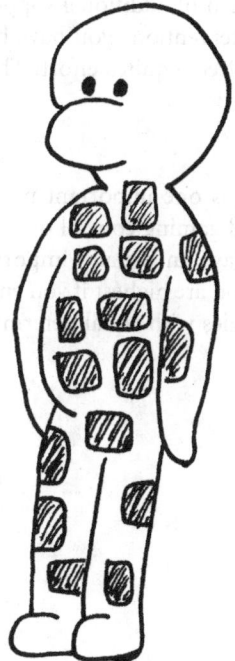

How *not* to use nicotine patches!

and inhaler are licensed (at the time of writing in the UK only) to be used concurrently with reducing the amount of smoking for a period of up to six weeks, and then for a further period of up to six months, if the smoker continues to cut down on consumption until smoke free. Use of NRT *without* concurrent smoking then continues from 6 to 9 months, with the aim to stop using NRT within 12 months. This procedure is known as the *Cut down then stop* (CDTS) approach.

Smoking while using bupropion is only "OK" in the first week of treatment, with a firm target stop date set by the second week of treatment. Within two weeks of starting to take the tablets, you must stop smoking.

Can nicotine replacement or bupropion make me stop smoking?

No! *You* are the only one who can make you stop smoking. None of these products alone offers a magical "cure" for your smoking habit. Remember, change comes from you being committed to doing things differently! Almost all evidence for the effectiveness of these products was found when they were used together with some form of additional support such as counseling and the cognitive–behavioral interventions you have been learning about in this program. Becoming smoke free requires effort! There is no magic bullet!

Putting it all together

Kicking the chemical habit is one important part of becoming smoke free. Doing things differently and gaining control over the behaviors and routines that support your habit plays an equally important role. Your chances of becoming smoke free for good are highest if you engage in both the behavioral and pharmacological strategies with equal determination and effort.

6

Staying smoke free I: enhancing motivation for change

THERAPIST GUIDELINES

Aims

1 Review which motivational challenges are relevant to which treatment phase
2 Explain the *Motivational worksheet*
3 Boost motivation in group members by matching different types of skill training to different motivational tasks: *initiating* change, *maintaining* change, *re-engaging* in change after a setback
4 Apply the principles of motivational interviewing to help group members to increase readiness for change, engage in change behaviors, and take responsibility for putting change into action
5 Discuss the role of reward.

In the assessment interview (Chapter 2), the baseline level of motivation for change for each group member was assessed in terms of *confidence* to achieve change, *readiness* to change, and *ambivalence* about change. These aspects of the change process need to be monitored throughout treatment and are discussed with clients early in the program, and then again whenever clients show signs that their motivation is wavering, or when clients enter a different phase of their change process (e.g., after quit day). The overall treatment plan and flexible use of individual treatment modules allows for a tailored response to the waxing and waning of motivation. The modules are designed to match the training of particular skills to the specific motivational challenges encountered at particular points in the change cycle along the continuum of readiness to change. Figure 6.1 provides an overview of the three types of motivation and skills involved in becoming smoke free for good.

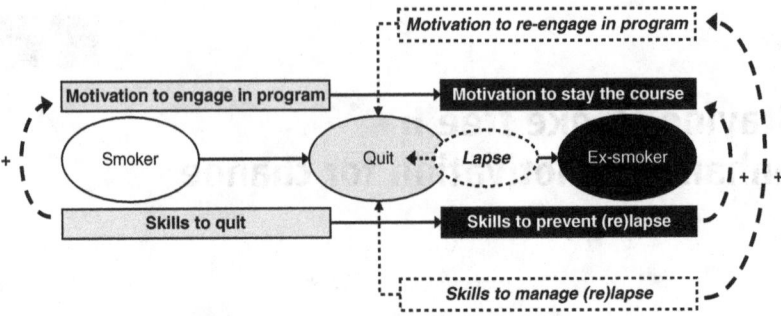

Figure 6.1 Types of motivation and skills in becoming smoke free.

Motivation to initiate engagement with the smoking cessation program

At the start of the group, it is essential to strengthen the clients' *motivation to engage in the program.* Change comes from doing things differently; if clients do not start doing things differently, you can guarantee that things will stay the same! Therefore, it is essential that clients from day one of the program engage in at least some of the behavioral change strategies introduced in the first group session (see *Client materials: How do I know when I need to "boost" my motivation?* for early warning signs that motivation may be wavering as the program gets under way). These behavioral strategies, along with practice in visualizing life as a non-smoker with the help of imagery exercises, are part of the skills training introduced in the first week of the program to move smokers in the direction of change. Any move in the right direction, however subtle (e.g., reduction in daily cigarette intake by 10% in the first week, and then again a similar amount in the second week), will be a confidence builder. That is, a client's sense of self-efficacy, or his or her belief that they can execute the desired behavior, is strengthened by learning skills helpful in executing that behavior (i.e., quitting). This confidence in their own skills to control at least some aspects of their smoking behavior can, in turn, increase clients' motivation to commit to a quit day soon thereafter (shown in Figure 6.1 by the "+" sign next to the broken arrow going from the *skills to quit* box to the corresponding *motivation to engage in program* box).

Motivation to maintain the change

Following quit day, the second type of motivation is targeted, the *motivation to stay the course.* As explained in the *Client materials* for this chapter, the key to *initiating* change is that clients expect that the benefits of changing will clearly outweigh the cost of making that change happen. In contrast, the key to *sustaining* change and reducing vulnerability to relapse is that clients experience some satisfaction with the progress they have made (Rothman, 2000). Therefore, to enhance motivation to stay the course, clients need to be encouraged during this phase to monitor how the transition to being a non-smoker has improved (a) how they feel, (b) their ability to do things they were not able to do as a smoker, and (c) the quality of interactions with significant others (*Client materials* has examples). In parallel, skills training will focus on the prevention of relapse. Practicing the skills of monitoring positive lifestyle changes and rehearsing relapse-prevention strategies increases clients' confidence that they are capable of doing what it takes to stay the course, which, in turn, can boost their motivation to put in the effort to apply these strategies (Figure 6.1).

Motivation to re-engage in the change process following a setback

As illustrated in Figure 6.1, the third type of motivation relevant to successful change, *the motivation to re-engage in the program*, comes into play after a setback has occurred. Most group members will have experienced the repeated cycling through the phases of quitting and relapsing typical of the recovery from addictive behaviors such as smoking (see the diagram of *The change cycle: steps to becoming smoke free* in the *Client materials*, which is based on Prochaska, DiClemente, & Norcross, 1992). It is important to communicate to clients that a lapse or relapse is quite normal and, therefore, not unexpected (Chapter 7 defines "lapse" and "relapse"). Enhancing motivation to re-engage in the treatment program after a setback involves preparation of the clients so that they understand that, when they are faced with a setback, (a) they must not give up; (b) they must not dwell on the slip but focus on the gains made prior to the setback; and (c) they must not view the lapse as a failure but rather as a learning opportunity for what to do better the next time. The specific skills to manage (re)lapse once it has occurred, and to minimize the likelihood of relapse occurring in the future, are both covered in Module 5, which is discussed in Chapter 7.

The change cycle: wheel of despair or exit strategy?

Note that the *Client materials* start with an illustration of the change cycle (Prochaska *et al.*, 1992). Begin the segment on motivation enhancement by discussing with clients the change cycle. This is a good lead into the topic because most clients will readily identify with the experience illustrated by the change cycle. It is always easier to get clients engaged in a topic if the starting point is something that is familiar to them from their personal experience. In talking about the change cycle, this is an opportunity to get several points across.

- Express empathic understanding of how hard and frustrating it must have been in the past to have tried and slipped back into old habits.
- Reassure clients that this is normal when trying to beat an addiction.
- Encourage clients to use their understanding of the change cycle to their advantage. That means, tell them that they need to be on guard to avoid falling into the motivational trap of viewing the change cycle as a "wheel of despair." Instead, focus their attention on to the parts of the change cycle that show a clear "exit strategy."
- Tell clients that they need to focus on two things when a setback occurs. First, do not let a slip be an excuse for giving up, and second, take a direct shortcut back into the action and maintenance steps. In practice this means, "come back to the next group session and get back on track." "Get straight back into the program, and let the group help you with renewing your effort and consolidate the changes you had made so far."
- Emphasize that the program offers all the tools and support to exit the change cycle successfully, but it is the *responsibility of each client* to use the tools and follow the exit strategy.
- Encourage clients to share with the group examples of times when they had a relapse in the past and may have not had the resolve to get right back onto the path toward action and maintenance. Ask about how they felt at the time. Expect to hear confessions of how they felt embarrassed, ashamed, or guilty for having failed. Use this as an opportunity to point out that these feelings are normal following a lapse, and that clients need to be wary of them because they are a common reason why people may not want to come back to the group anymore. They feel embarrassed and discouraged and want to avoid facing the other group members after their slip. It is very important to let them know that the group is not about judging people, it is about helping group members to succeed with their efforts in the long run. The group will not be disappointed that someone had a slip (because that is to be expected along the way to become smoke free). Instead, the group will welcome back with open arms anyone who had a lapse. The group will only be disappointed if a member after a slip decides not to come back to the group. The message to get across to the group members here is: be prepared that you might feel embarrassed and guilty after a setback, but do not seek comfort in avoidance; seek comfort from your fellow group members who understand exactly what you are going through. As mentioned above, the specific skills to manage (re)lapse once it has occurred, and to minimize the likelihood of relapse occurring in the future, are both covered later in the program (Module 5, discussed in Chapter 7). In this early session, the aim is to lay the

groundwork for helping clients to shift their understanding of a lapse. A lapse is not to be viewed as an insurmountable roadblock signaling the end of the journey, but rather as a temporary detour with the ultimate goal of being smoke free still clear ahead. Reframing relapse in this way early in the program helps to diffuse its potential for later undermining the motivation to stay the course.

Understanding ambivalence

After explaining how to use a better understanding of the change cycle to mobilize motivational energy to anticipate and overcome setbacks while keeping the momentum going in the direction of the exit window in the cycle, it is important to raise clients' awareness of another motivational trap that can keep clients stuck in their old ways. That is, the exit strategy often gets stalled in ambivalence (Miller, 1998). Understanding and resolving ambivalence is a key in eliciting change and is a central aim of motivational interviewing (Miller & Rollnick, 2002). Therefore, the second section in the *Client materials* on how to enhance motivation for change encourages clients to view ambivalence as something positive. While ambivalence can lead to indecision and inaction, it also represents a window of opportunity (see the diagram in the *Client materials* on *Motivational balance space*, which is adapted from Stritzke *et al.* (2007).). As explained in Chapter 2, the process of moving a client from feeling not ambivalent about their smoking to feeling ambivalent about it is referred to as "developing a discrepancy." Clients are encouraged to explore how their current behavior as a smoker is incompatible with their desire to enjoy the benefits they envisage that life as a non-smoker will give them. Once a discrepancy becomes clear to clients, the next step is to amplify the importance of the desired goals or values relative to the importance of continuing to smoke. This is done by facilitating clients' self-exploration of what the things are that keep them stalled in ambivalence, and what the things are that can get them unstuck and strengthen their resolve to tip the motivational balance in favor of change. It is important that the client rather than the group facilitators present the arguments for change (Miller & Rollnick, 2002). The *Motivational worksheet* in the *Client materials* is designed to help with that task. Consider the example of a client who has had repeated heart bypass surgery and was told by his doctor that another heart attack would most certainly be fatal. Although for many people this threat of an imminent death would be motivation enough to quit smoking, this "cost" in the left column of his motivational worksheet was not sufficient to tip the balance toward change for *him*. What ultimately made the difference for this client was his daughter's refusal to visit him with his young grandchildren, because she did not want to expose them to second-hand smoke. It was the benefits of enjoying time with his grandchildren in his retirement, not the high risk of a premature death from his smoking, that prompted him to cross the motivational threshold and quit for good.

The motivational worksheet

The *Motivational worksheet* in the *Client materials* is divided into four sections. The two sections in the left column (benefits of being smoke free and costs of continuing to smoke) are used to list things that strengthen motivation for change. The two sections in the right column (benefits of continuing to smoke and costs of becoming smoke free) are used to list things that weaken motivation for change. Before coming to the group, smokers typically will have already thought a lot about the things in the left column. That is, thinking about the costs of smoking and the benefits of not smoking would have prompted their decision to join a smoking cessation program. In contrast, smokers generally are less aware of, or have often not explicitly considered, the things in the right column. But it is those things in the right column that often undermine smokers' motivation for change and keep them stuck in their old, unhealthy ways. When introducing the worksheet to clients, the following steps are helpful in getting clients to engage with the task and start generating their own views of what they perceive as the cost and benefits of quitting versus not quitting.

- Begin by explaining the four sections of the worksheet. Point out that the right column contains important things that smokers often have not really thought much about, because they are deliberately trying to *not* focus on the things that they find appealing about smoking. Point out that it is very important to pay attention to the things in the right column, because those things are barriers to change.
- Distribute the worksheet to group members and ask them to think for a moment and write at least one or two things in each section in the left column. It is good to start with the left column, because most smokers find it easier to come up with things to list in the left column. Then ask clients to tell the other group members what they have put down in each section. List the group's contributions on an overhead or whiteboard. Then do the same with the right column.
- Encourage discussion about similarities and differences among the things listed and how they might strengthen or weaken each member's motivation for change. Ask what group members plan to do to minimize the impact of the things in the right column so that they do not undermine their efforts.
- Point out that if they can come up with more things in the left column than in the right column, that is a good position to be in. But it is critical also to point out that it is not a simple bean-counting exercise; just putting more

things in the left column may not be enough to tip the motivational balance toward change. It matters not only *how many* items are in each column, but *how important* (!) each item is. For example, a single item in the right column can be so important to a client that even a dozen "good reasons" in the left column do not make up for the personal importance attached to the one item in the opposite column.

- After discussion of the few examples generated in this group exercise, ask the group members to use the worksheet at home and generate as many items for themselves as they can think of to put in their own personal worksheet. Ask them to bring their completed worksheet to the next group session, so that you can make copies of them for further discussion and treatment planning. Doing this exercise is useful both in terms of *outcome* and in terms of *process*. The outcome will help with personalizing treatment plans for each group member. The process can help to identify clients who are unwilling to make the commitment in time and energy to do change work on their own between sessions. The latter in itself may signal the need for intensifying motivation-boosting interventions for those group members.

FRAMES: six active ingredients of interventions to enhance motivation

There are a number of intervention strategies found to be effective in enhancing motivation for change. These can be organized under the acronym FRAMES: feedback, responsibility, advice, menu, empathy, and self-efficacy (Miller, 1995).

F: Feedback

The information gathered in the structured assessment interview prior to the first group session is used to give each client *personalized* feedback about the harm and negative consequences of their smoking behavior. For example, clients are given the *Carbon monoxide (CO) monitoring information sheet* together with their own personal *Carbon monoxide (CO) feedback chart*. The loss of income through financing the smoking habit will be highlighted based on the data collected in the interview. Other consequences relevant to a given client such as health risks for themselves or others exposed to secondary smoke from the client's habit will be summarized and fed back to each client. In one of the early modules (Module 2: *The ins and outs of becoming smoke free* [discussed in Ch. 4]), the negative effects associated with smoking in terms of acute short-term and long-term health risks, and in terms of social and interpersonal disadvantages, will be reviewed. Group discussion will relate those negative effects to the personal circumstances of each client. When giving this personal feedback, be mindful of two principles:

- give feedback in a matter-of-fact voice and tone; avoid dramatizing and scare-mongering
- give feedback regularly; use the weekly monitoring data to update personal feedback, making sure to highlight positive gains as well as evidence of setbacks or stagnation in the client's change efforts.

R: Responsibility

A key ingredient of effective motivational interventions is putting emphasis on the clients' personal responsibility for their own change and the fact that it is up to them to make choices about their behavior. The message is simple: "No one can change your smoking for you; it's up to you to make the change. You can choose to keep on smoking as you have been, or you can choose to do things differently. Here are the tools, but it is up to you to use them." Clients who perceive that they have a choice in the matter are more likely to accept responsibility to engage in the change process, embrace the change strategies, and persist with the effort needed to put them into action.

A: Advice

Although motivation to become smoke free is often high in people who have taken the step of joining a smoking cessation program, most smokers do not have clear ideas about how and when they might quit (Herzog & Blagg, 2007). Giving each client clear and direct advice as to the need for change and how it can be accomplished is a simple strategy to enhance the momentum for change. Such "hands-on" recommendations provide a motivational boost that capitalizes on the readiness of the client to give it a go by "coaching" clients on how to embark on a personal and workable change plan (Miller & Rollnick, 2002). Giving advice and coaching clients on how to translate their motivation into action is not to be confused with ordering or pressuring clients to do something. Giving advice involves making clear recommendations for change in an empathic manner while acknowledging that each client is responsible for making the ultimate choice and managing their own change plan.

M: Menu

If clients are to take responsibility for making choices about their own change plan, they must be offered alternatives from among which they can choose. The *Behavioral changes chart* (introduced in the first group session, Module 1, which is discussed in Chapter 3) offers a menu of options from which the clients can select those change strategies that they are most ready to tackle first. Providing a menu of options also has the function of lowering the threshold for making the first active step in the direction of change. With so many options to choose from, surely each client can find something that is "doable" for them. With a menu of options, clients will run out of excuses why they "can't do this right now." In this way, the menu helps to overcome inaction by making the first step toward change easier. The principle of a menu of options is also used for other key elements of the treatment program. When clients make choices about using pharmacotherapy to aid with their quit attempt, they can select from a number of equally effective alternatives based on their personal preferences (Chapter 5). Similarly, the group program does not require adherence to a pre-set quit day. Rather, a window of opportunity (after about four weeks into the program) is recommended as a time period within which clients can choose to set a personal quit day. Again, the scheduling of a quit day is personalized in accordance with the principles that (a) clients are responsible for their change and have a choice, (b) therapists provide clear advice and recommendations about what time-frame for setting a quit day is most advantageous, and (c) there is a menu of alternative time points that individual clients can choose from.

E: Empathy

Adoption of an empathic communication style is very effective in enhancing motivation for change. An empathic style involves being warm, supportive, sympathetic, and attentive. Less helpful is a style that is overly directive, confrontational, aggressive, and suspicious. An empathic group facilitator is one who accepts the clients' efforts without criticism or blame. As mentioned above, clear directions are provided in a gentle, respectful, "coaching" manner, rather than in a coercive, pushy fashion. Reflective listening strategies help to gain an empathic understanding of the smoker's experience. It involves being attentive and hearing what a group member is saying and feeling, making a guess to the meaning of what one has just heard, and then communicating this understanding back to the client with a statement. For example, a client may state that he wants to quit smoking cigarettes but still wants to smoke an occasional joint because he feels that helps him to stay more relaxed when dealing with a current conflict with his in-laws. Empathy for his situation might be expressed by stating, "It can be very difficult to make two major changes at once, quitting cigarettes and stopping smoking marijuana. You sound quite stressed and overwhelmed by having to deal with these family issues at the same time." This empathic response to the client's predicament could be followed up with offering the client a choice to learn more about alternative ways of dealing with this type of stressful interpersonal conflict by stating, "It is common that smokers find it more difficult to quit when dealing with stressful personal circumstances like yours. That's why we have a few handouts on problem-solving skills that can help clients to learn alternative strategies to cope with situations like yours without resorting to smoking. This way, this big stress that's going on in your life right now does not undermine your efforts to become smoke free." And then, directed to the group as a whole, one could ask: "Do you think it might be helpful if we gave each of you a couple of handouts that provide you with hints and strategies on how to make stressful situations more manageable without choosing smoking as your 'coping crutch'? We can then discuss those strategies in more detail next time." In sum, communicating empathy with the client's predicament can be combined with the other elements of motivational interviewing of advice giving and offering choice to enhance motivation for change.

S: Self-efficacy

Self-efficacy refers to the smoker's belief or self-confidence that she or he can carry out the tasks required to become smoke free. Smokers will not consider change unless they think it is possible. Optimism in one's ability to change sustains motivation and effort. Acquiring additional skills increases one's sense that one can take on tasks that initially appear very difficult. Enhancing motivation for smoking cessation, therefore, goes hand in hand with the training of specific skills (Figure 6.1). Several strategies are particularly helpful in increasing self-efficacy in clients.

- The use of the *Behavioral change chart* to monitor the clients' progress with making changes to their everyday smoking-related routines can provide a big motivational boost to clients. Once they see that changes they have made led to a direct change (even if only small to begin with) in the number of cigarettes smoked or their carbon monoxide readings, they experience a sense of control over their behavior. Breaking down the more distant goal of becoming a non-smoker into smaller steps provides clients with opportunities to experience partial successes along the way. Experiencing success with setting more proximal goals and achieving them is a big confidence builder before getting ready to take the bigger step of quitting for good.
- The group facilitator's own optimism can influence client motivation. Expressing confidence in the clients' ability to change goes a long way in bolstering client self-efficacy. This takes the form of acting as both coach and cheerleader while communicating the message "You can do it!" All new learning is made easier when strong support is readily available.
- In particular, self-efficacy can receive a big boost with the ongoing support and encouragement of the other group members. This is one of the key advantages of group treatment over individual treatment. It is, therefore, important that the therapists regularly foster opportunities for these group

processes to occur. Similarly, clients should be encouraged to assist other members in mastering the skills applied in the program. Helping others with a particular skill strengthens one's own mastery in that skill and hence solidifies and further builds one's own self-efficacy.

- Social support outside of the group can also boost self-efficacy for becoming smoke free. If feasible, clients may find a "buddy" who can help them with maintaining change behaviors or by providing a non-smoking context for problem solving. For example, a buddy might agree to go for a walk every night after dinner to disrupt a client's routine of smoking after a meal. A buddy may also serve as a personal "helpline" to be contacted by phone if a client feels they are about to stray from their change plan.
- Preparation and practice for what to do when encountering situations that constitute a high risk for relapse can build self-efficacy (Chapter 7).
- Learning how to implement stress-management strategies and problem-solving skills during the challenging period of becoming smoke free increases self-efficacy. Guidelines and client materials for that purpose are provided in Chapter 8 (Module 6 on *Staying smoke free III: coping without smoking*) and Chapter 9 (Module 7 on *Thoughts: how they affect smoking behaviors*).

The role of reward

For most people, being rewarded for one's efforts is a powerful motivator to keep up the good work. Many clients in our groups have found it helpful to set up a reward system for themselves. The *Client materials* provide a few examples of what types of reward system clients in previous groups have used to motivate themselves. These are not meant as prescriptions of what clients are to do, but as ideas that can stimulate clients to come up with their own ways of rewarding their change behaviors along the way.

Tips for working with individuals

The treatment objectives of this module apply when working with individuals in the same way as they do for group interventions. Only minor adjustments need to be made when following the therapist guidelines.

In the section on introducing the *Change cycle*, the important message that needs to be communicated to the client still is that the key is to come back to the next session in the event of a lapse, and get back on track. But some of the tips on how to take advantage of the group as a support network to help with renewing the client's change effort and consolidating the gains made prior to the lapse are not applicable in the one-on-one

Tips (cont.)

context. It is up to the therapist to provide that supporting role. Although the group support is lost in individual interventions, there is a trade-off. A client may find it less embarrassing to return to treatment after a slip-up when he or she only needs to "face-up" to the therapist rather than to a whole group of fellow clients.

In the section providing guidance on how to work with the *Motivational worksheet*, the following in the bulleted list of steps can be slightly adapted for the one-on-one context.

- When eliciting one or two things to be entered in the columns of the worksheet, this will obviously only be done once (rather than asking each group member). But it is still useful to transfer all worksheet entries, even if generated only by a single client, onto a whiteboard. This has the effect of bringing the client's private thoughts out in the open and subjecting them to honest scrutiny and further elaboration. Because some clients initially may have difficulty in generating a number of items for each quadrant of the worksheet without the collective effort from others, as in the group context, the onus is on the therapist actively to encourage the client to produce a number of items in each of the worksheet quadrants. The therapist can make this task easier for the client by asking him or her to just jot down a "quick list" of items for each quadrant, and leave discussion of the items and what they mean in relation to the client's journey to become smoke free for after the worksheet has been completed.
- As the worksheet entries are only from one client, there is no discussion of similarities and differences among the things listed by different group members. Rather, the session can proceed directly to asking the client what she or he plans to do to minimize the things in the right column so that they do not undermine the change efforts.
- Because it is important in the group context to involve all group members when introducing the worksheet activity, time constraints only permit each member to generate one or two items for each quadrant. Then, after discussion of the collated "group worksheet," clients are instructed to generate further items on their own as a homework assignment. When working with only one client, there is sufficient time to complete this task directly in the session with the therapist's guidance.

In the section explaining the FRAMES approach to *motivational interviewing*, some aspects unique to the group context can be omitted or streamlined when working with individuals.

F: Feedback. There will be no group discussion of the different profiles that link the smoking behaviors and associate harm and negative

Tips (cont.)

consequences to the particular circumstances of each client. Instead, the focus is directly on the personalized feedback for the individual client.

E: Empathy. If it becomes relevant to offer the option of including in the treatment program the modules on problem solving or stress management, the guidelines show how in the group context one can go about gaining the cooperation from the group as a whole to add these modules to the treatment program to accommodate the needs of some of the group members. This usually requires some sensitivity toward maintaining a balance between the different needs of individual group members and attention to building strong rapport with the group and among its members. An advantage of working with only one client is that responding flexibly to the particular needs of that client is straightforward and can be integrated in the treatment plan without consideration of other clients.

S: Self-efficacy. Some parts of the bulleted list of strategies to increase self-efficacy in clients must be omitted or modified when working with individuals. Obviously, the mutual support inherent in group treatments cannot be recruited to facilitate skill acquisition and boost self-efficacy. Therefore, the guidelines on boosting self-efficacy with the help of social support outside the group become even more important in the context of one-on-one interventions.

Finally, with respect to the *Client materials,* clients are encouraged to monitor any changes in their daily smoking routines and the benefits that stem from those changes. In the group context, clients are encouraged to share these experiences with the other group members at each session. Although clients in the one-on-one treatment context do not have the benefit of comparing notes with fellow clients on what works and what does not in making progress toward becoming smoke free, individual clients can be instructed to ignore the few lines referring specifically to groups in the client handout and share their experiences with the therapist instead.

CLIENT MATERIALS

1 The change cycle: steps to becoming smoke free
2 Motivation for change: how to make motivation strong and keep it up.

The change cycle: steps to becoming smoke free

The cycle of quitting and relapsing is only too familiar to smokers attempting to quit. Many go through the steps of thinking about quitting, doing something about it, managing without cigarettes for a while, and then returning to their previous level of smoking several times before they stay smoke free for good. The solid arrows in the diagram below show the steps that represent progress toward the goal of becoming smoke free. The dashed arrows indicate setbacks.

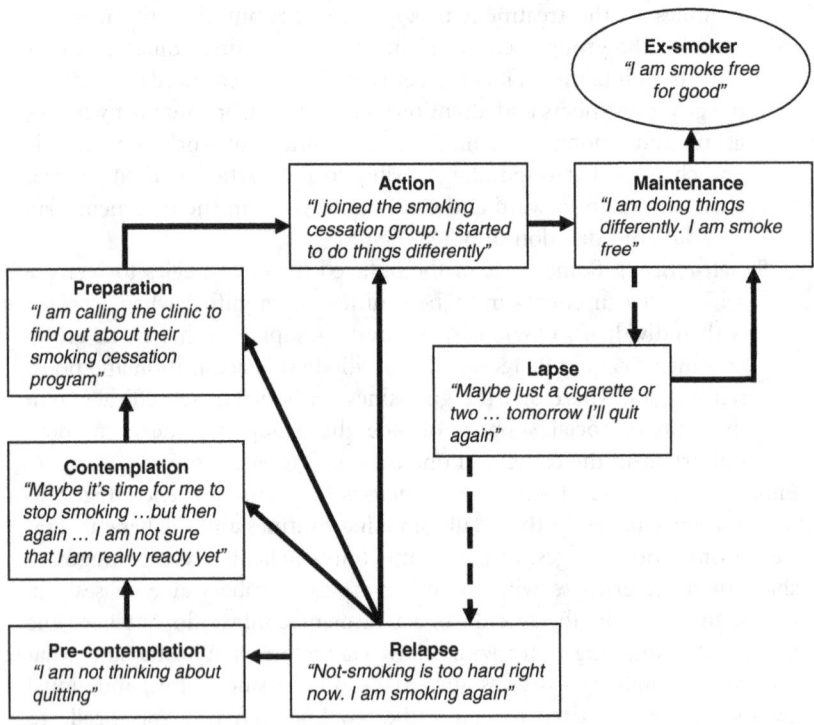

With the help of the smoking cessation group you have joined, you will learn strategies and skills that make it easier to break free from this cycle and become an ex-smoker. Importantly, there are direct shortcuts back to the action and maintenance steps in case you have a "slip" along the way. Needless to say, this is not meant as permission to have a lapse whenever you feel like it. Rather, it means that if you do have a lapse, do not give up! You can learn from your lapse and then take responsibility for going straight back to the smoke-free path. This will bring you closer to being an ex-smoker.

Motivation for change: how to make motivation strong and keep it up

Becoming smoke free has many rewards, but getting there requires effort. To put in the right amount of effort, you need to be motivated. You need to have strong enough motivation initially to put change into motion by beginning to do things differently. This is hard because it is always easier to do the things one is used to than to try out new ways of doing things. Once you have started to put in the effort to make changes that will disrupt your daily routines as a smoker and move you toward a non-smoking lifestyle, you need again strong motivation to put in the hard work to maintain those changes. That is, you need to keep practicing those new ways of doing things until they are so familiar that they have become part of your everyday life and require little effort.

Understanding ambivalence

Motivation for change is not all or none. It is common among smokers who have joined a smoking cessation program to experience some ambivalence toward making such a profound lifestyle change. While your desire to *not* smoke was a strong motivating force in prompting you to join a smoking cessation group, this does not mean that your desire to *still* smoke has all of a sudden vanished into thin air. Ambivalence, or feeling two ways about something, is not a bad state to be in. In fact, ambivalence is good for you, because it means that you have moved from acceptance of yourself as a smoker, who gives little serious thought to becoming a non-smoker, to questioning your choice of being a smoker. As shown in the diagram below, ambivalence is a normal step toward becoming a non-smoker. As your desire to *avoid* smoking increases in strength, it provides a counterweight to the strong automatic pattern of still wanting to smoke. Once your desire to avoid smoking becomes more practiced and remains strong, and urges to smoke weaken in the weeks after quitting, the motivational balance tips in favor of not-smoking, making it easier to consolidate the change in lifestyle you have made.

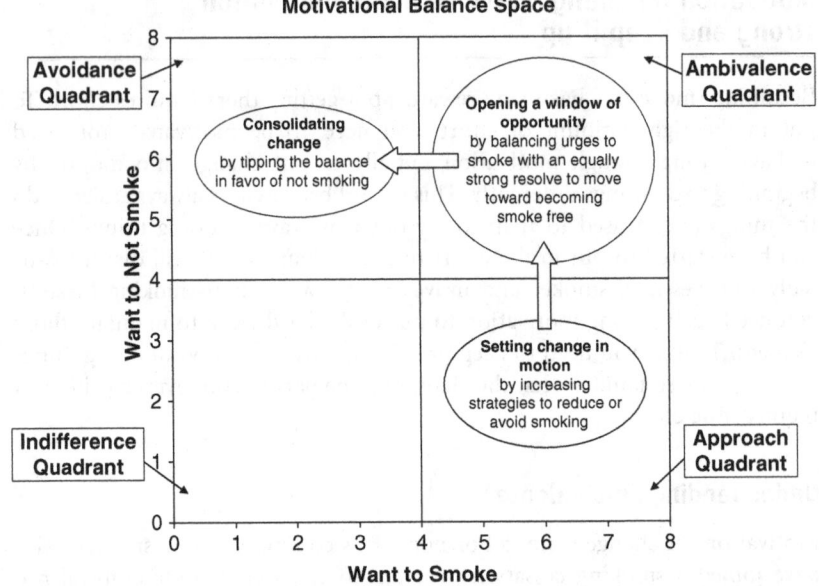

Motivational Balance Space

How do I strengthen my motivation for change?

Feeling ambivalent is like having two voices inside you that compete for your attention: The "no" voice says "I want to *not* smoke anymore" and the "yes" voice says, "I really want a cigarette right now." You can strengthen your motivation for change in two ways. First, by generating as many arguments as you can for the voice that helps you to avoid smoking. Second, by knowing your "enemy." That is, list all the arguments that your "yes" voice uses to convince you that this is not really a good time to quit smoking. There are benefits that smokers often believe they get from smoking (e.g., "Smoking calms my nerves when I am stressed"), and there could be costs, at least temporarily, associated with quitting (e.g., "Two of my best friends are smoking ... if I go out with them, it will be hard not to relapse, so I may have to stay away from them for a while"). Use the *Motivational worksheet* to list the arguments put forward by the voice that supports your goal of quitting, and the voice that wants you to stay the same.

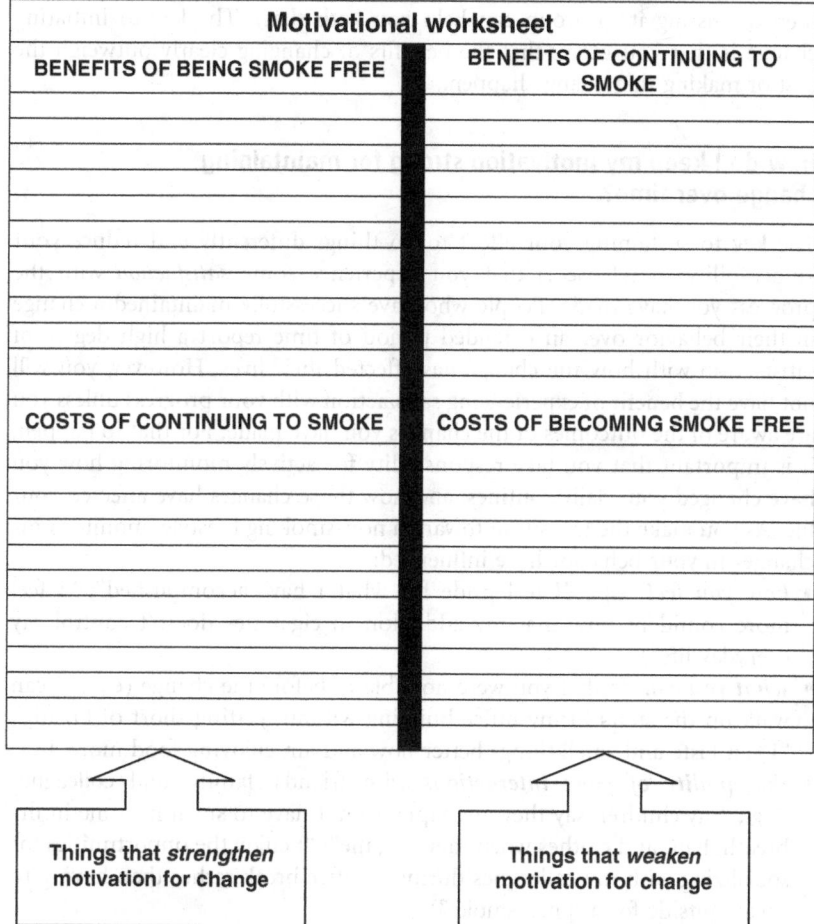

Motivational worksheet

BENEFITS OF BEING SMOKE FREE	BENEFITS OF CONTINUING TO SMOKE

COSTS OF CONTINUING TO SMOKE	COSTS OF BECOMING SMOKE FREE

Things that *strengthen* motivation for change

Things that *weaken* motivation for change

How do I know when I need to "boost" my motivation?

By coming along to a smoking cessation group, you obviously were motivated enough to invest time and energy into improving your health and overall well-being. One of the first warning signs that your motivation may be wavering early in your attempt to become smoke free is *if you do not start to do things differently* but chose to put off using any of the behavioral change strategies introduced in the first group session. All the strategies listed on the behavioral changes chart are simple and do not require special skills to put into action. If you find yourself going a whole week without even applying a single one of those strategies on a regular basis, then you need to take an honest look at what holds you back (filling out the *Motivational worksheet* and then discussing it in group can help you with that). The key to initiating change is that you *expect* that the benefits of changing clearly outweigh the cost of making that change happen.

How do I keep my motivation strong for maintaining change over time?

The key to sustaining your effort to do things differently and reduce your vulnerability to relapse is that you experience some *satisfaction* with the progress you have made. People who have successfully maintained a change in their behavior over an extended period of time report a high degree of satisfaction with how the change has affected their lives. However, you will not have the benefit of experiencing satisfaction with your progress unless you are aware of the outcomes of the changes you have made. For that to happen, it is important that you take responsibility for actively monitoring how you have changed your daily routines, and how those changes have affected your life. As you make the transition toward a non-smoking lifestyle, monitor how changes in your behavior have influenced:

- *how you feel* (e.g., "I feel pride for what I have accomplished"; "I feel more confident now that my addiction to cigarettes doesn't control my everyday life")
- *what you can do* that you were not able to before the change (e.g., "I can walk up the stairs in my office building without getting short of breath"; "I can taste and smell things better now and am enjoying food more")
- *the quality of your interactions* with friends, family, and colleagues (e.g., "my children say they are happy to not have to smell nicotine in my breath, hair, and clothes when they hug me"; "I enjoy the opportunities for socializing with my colleagues during a coffee break rather than having to sneak outside for a quick smoke").

It is a good idea to take note of these changes on a weekly basis and share them with the other members in the smoking cessation group. Comparing notes with the group helps to raise awareness of benefits that may have gone unnoticed or be taken for granted otherwise. It also helps to encourage group members whose motivation may have been wavering after a lapse.

It is also helpful for keeping your motivation high if you *express* your satisfaction with the progress you are making by celebrating it! For most people, being rewarded for one's efforts is a powerful motivator to keep up the good work. Many clients in our groups have found it helpful to set up a reward system for themselves. For example, you may start off with something small, such as rewarding yourself with a sticker for each day that you are actively engaging in change strategies. When you have reached a certain number of stickers, treat yourself (e.g., movie, new CD, a massage). Or, some like to draw up a progress chart where you can mark off the amount of money you save each week from not buying cigarettes. Some clients even collected money in a jar from the cigarettes that they did not smoke, and kept it in a prominent place in their home as a concrete reminder of how they are changing. You will be surprised how quickly it all adds up. By celebrating your new lifestyle changes in this way, you are making sure that you are not taking them for granted, and this will increase your satisfaction with what you have accomplished.

7

Staying smoke free II: prevention and management of a lapse or relapse

THERAPIST GUIDELINES

Aims

1 Review the distinction between a lapse and relapse
2 Assist clients in identifying high-risk situations
3 Coach clients in strategies for the effective management of high-risk situations, including stimulus control, smoking-refusal skills, and coping with withdrawal distress and cravings
4 Manage setbacks by reframing "lapse" as a temporary setback and a window of opportunity for learning, rather than as the end of the quit attempt and failure.

The *Client materials* for this module begin with an explanation of the distinction between a "lapse" and a "relapse." A lapse refers to smoking one or a few cigarettes after at least 24 hours of abstinence followed by a resumption of the quit attempt, and relapse is the return to regular smoking, even if at a lower level than prior to the quit attempt. We recommend that group facilitators introduce these definitions with clients already in Module 4 (covered in Ch. 6) when discussing the change cycle, and then review them at the start of the session introducing the current module on relapse management. There have been attempts to standardize the duration of a lapse period (no more than six consecutive days) before it becomes a relapse (more than six consecutive days), but other thresholds for duration and number of cigarettes smoked have also been used (Curry & McBride, 1994). However, these precise thresholds remain largely arbitrary and do not do justice to the dynamic nature of the lapse/relapse process (Brandon, Vidrine, & Litvin, 2007). Nicotine addiction is a chronic, relapsing disorder where neither periods of abstinence nor relapse are viewed as final outcomes but rather as progress data, which inform decisions about adjustments to the treatment plan. This module presents the

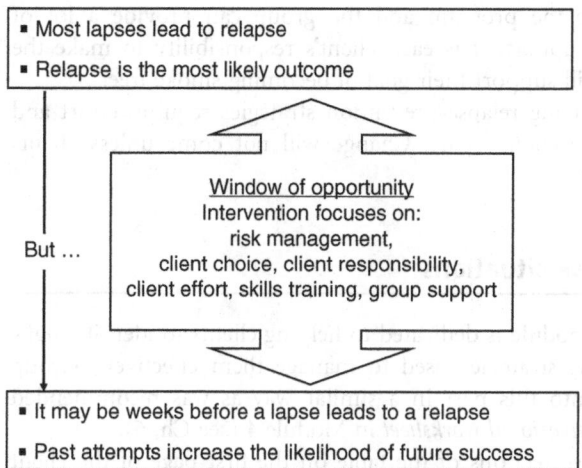

Figure 7.1 A window of opportunity for managing lapses.

strategies used during the phase of the treatment plan when clients have commenced a smoke-free episode. Hence, it is typically introduced around the time that some of the group members have chosen as their quit date.

The importance of actively engaging clients in relapse prevention and management is illustrated in Figure 7.1. It is a sobering statistic of smoking cessation attempts that relapse is the most likely outcome and that most lapses lead to relapse (Piasecki, 2006). The good news is that there is often a delay between an initial lapse and a full return to regular smoking (Dodgen, 2005), and previous attempts increase the likelihood of future success (e.g., Yzer & van den Putte, 2006). This provides a window of opportunity for engaging clients in intervention strategies that facilitate their re-engagement with the treatment program and a swift resumption of their quit attempt.

Reviewing the distinction between a lapse and relapse

When discussing the distinction between a lapse and relapse at the beginning of this session, it is helpful to emphasize the following points.

- Referring back to the group discussion of the change cycle in an earlier session, state that this session is about learning how to make a lapse less likely to occur and, in the event it should happen, how to avoid letting it derail the clients' goal of becoming smoke free.
- Reassure the clients that the program will give them the right tools to make the prevention and management of lapses easier.

- Reiterate that while the program and the group can provide a lot of practical help and support, it is each client's responsibility to make the right choices that will support their goal of becoming smoke free.
- Emphasize that applying relapse-prevention strategies requires effort and commitment on the clients' part. Change will not come unless clients actively (!) pursue it.

Identifying high-risk situations

The next part of this module is dedicated to helping clients to identify high-risk situations and the strategies used to manage them effectively. Group facilitators can lead into this part in a similar way as was recommended for explaining the *Motivational worksheet* in Module 4 (see Ch. 6).

First, explain the five sections of the table on the first page of the client handouts under *How do I prevent a lapse?*

Second, explain that knowing what is most likely to trip you up in your quit attempt is the first step of prevention.

Then go on to point out that the first two sections in the table are about emotionally stressful situations that can trigger a lapse. As is explained in the handout, these can be ongoing and may make it hard to come up with the energy to engage in the tasks associated with becoming smoke free. Or they may arise and peak at a particular moment, presenting an acute challenge that needs a fast and decisive response to contain the heightened relapse risk. The strategies used to manage these situations are not necessarily focused on smoking-related issues, but more broadly help clients to cope with difficult situations in their day-to-day lives. Group facilitators must be mindful that some clients may be reluctant to learn about these "counseling-type" strategies, as they prefer to focus on only those things directly related to their smoking behavior and quit attempt (i.e., the things listed in the last three sections of the table in the client handout). Other clients will readily want to take advantage of the opportunity to learn more about some of these general coping strategies, as they are keen to avoid letting such issues sabotage their quit attempt. This situation can be handled sensitively by (a) stating that the management strategies associated with the first two categories of high-risk situations are covered in a separate handout, and (b) asking if the group would like to learn about these in a subsequent session. Usually a consensus quickly emerges, and those group members who might have been reluctant have the option of scaling back their active participation during such a segment (although they may still benefit vicariously). When offering to cover this separate module, the group facilitators will already have a pretty good idea from the individual assessment interviews which clients would likely benefit most from covering some general coping skills training.

The next step is to shift the focus on to the last three sections of the table. Encourage clients to come up with some examples of high-risk situations from their own experience. Also, ask which of the associated management strategies they may have already used, and to what extent those strategies were helpful in the past. This serves two purposes. It identifies strategies that were helpful in the past and hence are more readily adopted again. It also identifies strategies that have not worked for a particular client. Some follow-up questioning might reveal inconsistent or incorrect use of the strategy. That information can be used to motivate clients to engage in those strategies again rather than making the premature assumption that a particular strategy "won't work for me."

After discussion of a few examples generated in this group exercise, ask the group members to take the worksheet entitled *My personal high-risk situations worksheet* home and to bring the completed sheet back to the next group session, so that the follow-up discussion can focus on the specific situations relevant to the members of this particular group.

Next we turn to coaching clients in the strategies for managing high-risk situations listed in the last three sections of the lapse prevention table.

Preparing for high-risk situations

Stimulus control

A good lead-in for this topic is to remind clients of the first session of the program, where clients learned that a powerful component of their nicotine addiction is the strong association of their smoking with cues linked to daily behavioral routines, people, and places. Ask clients to give some examples of cues in their environment that they strongly associate with smoking. Then ask them how confident they are that they would be able to resist the temptation to smoke if they were exposed to any of those triggers. Help clients problem solve by inviting discussion of the feasibility of (a) staying away altogether from those particular high-risk situations for a while, and (b) generating alternative means of enjoying the non-smoking-related benefits that clients normally derive from the situations they are better off avoiding for a while.

Smoking-refusal skills

When avoidance of high-risk social situations is not feasible, well-practiced smoking-refusal skills can help to manage these situations without giving in when offered a cigarette by someone else. This segment is best presented in three steps.

1 Using the client handout as a guide, briefly review the three general styles of refusal: passive, aggressive, and assertive. Explain how the three styles can either hinder or support the effectiveness of the refusal message.

2 Go over the three points in the handout explaining the elements of an assertive refusal, and then review the five simple strategies on what to do when someone offers the client a cigarette.

3 Model to the clients the three different ways of getting a refusal message across. Then, invite them to break up in pairs and practice these different ways with each other and provide supportive feedback. This exercise often generates quite a bit of humor among the group, but often leads clients to comment later how amazed they were that these little changes to their communications with other smokers made it so much easier to say "no."

Managing withdrawal distress

Smokers often cite the experience of unpleasant withdrawal symptoms as an excuse for weakening their resolve and having a lapse. The key message to get across here is that withdrawal symptoms are short lived! They peak in the first week and typically disappear within 10 days after smoking the last cigarette (Hughes, 2007; Shiffman et al., 2006). Those clients reporting strong withdrawal distress should be advised to consider using nicotine-replacement products, which are effective in reducing withdrawal symptoms (details on the use of these products are covered in Module 3, which is discussed in Chapter 5). A single session of exercise between 5 and 40 minutes can also effectively reduce withdrawal symptoms during the exercise and for up to 50 minutes after the exercise (Taylor, Ussher, & Faulkner, 2007).

Managing cravings

Most lapses are preceded by conscious cravings (Catley, O'Connell, & Shiffman, 2000). That is, cravings are not automatic processes that inevitably lead someone to an "absent-minded" lapse. Rather, cravings signal the need for making choices. They typically involve a conscious, effortful struggle between the desire for smoking a cigarette and a desire to remain abstinent (Stritzke et al., 2007; Tiffany, 1990). This is summarized in the client handout under *Managing cravings* as "six simple points to remember." Begin this segment by reviewing with the group these six points and emphasize that clients should view any experience of cravings as a signal to immediately begin engaging in actions and thoughts that are incompatible with and counteract any deliberate thoughts or behaviors designed to bring the client closer to obtaining a cigarette. The two figures in the client handout help to illustrate that craving management involves continuously making choices about whether to engage in behavioral steps and thoughts that assist in staying smoke free, or whether to take steps and make plans that weaken the resolve to remain smoke free.

End this segment by discussing the benefits of using a reminder card. Explain that the conscious struggle between wanting to give in to the craving and at the same time wanting to stay smoke free takes effort and it is often hard to think clearly in such situations. It is easier to know what to do in these situations before the voice in one's head that strongly argues to have a cigarette complicates matters. This is where the reminder card comes in. Just as an airline pilot in an emergency is trained to consult and follow a step-by-step emergency response manual (which minimizes the risk of making the wrong decisions under pressure), so a client can consult and follow his or her own personal craving response plan on the reminder card. Distribute index cards to the group members and ask them to write down the coping steps they want to engage in using the sample card in the client handout as a guide. Suggest that they write down helpful *actions* on the front of the card, and helpful *thoughts* on the back.

Managing setbacks

Whereas the previous parts in this module addressed strategies for preventing a lapse, the last part covers the situation when a lapse has happened. On a procedural note, depending on the number of clients in the group and their level of engagement with the discussion and practice of the prevention strategies, there may not be enough time in a single session also to cover the steps of what to do when a lapse occurs. This is not a problem because these topics can be introduced quite flexibly and are likely to be revisited repeatedly as clients will vary when they set their quit date and when they need help with rebounding from a lapse.

The aim of this segment is to reframe a lapse as a temporary setback and a window of opportunity for learning, rather than as the end of the quit attempt and failure. The key message to get across is that after a lapse clients should not give up, but return to the next group session and let the program help them to get back on track. The specific steps covered in the client handout are to (a) review what and how it happened, (b) make use of a step-by-step reminder card similar to the one used for dealing with cravings but with instructions on what to do following a lapse, (c) challenge unhelpful thinking, and (d) renew the commitment to be smoke free. Initially these steps are presented in a didactic manner as information on what to do after a lapse. Once a client returns to the group after experiencing a lapse, those

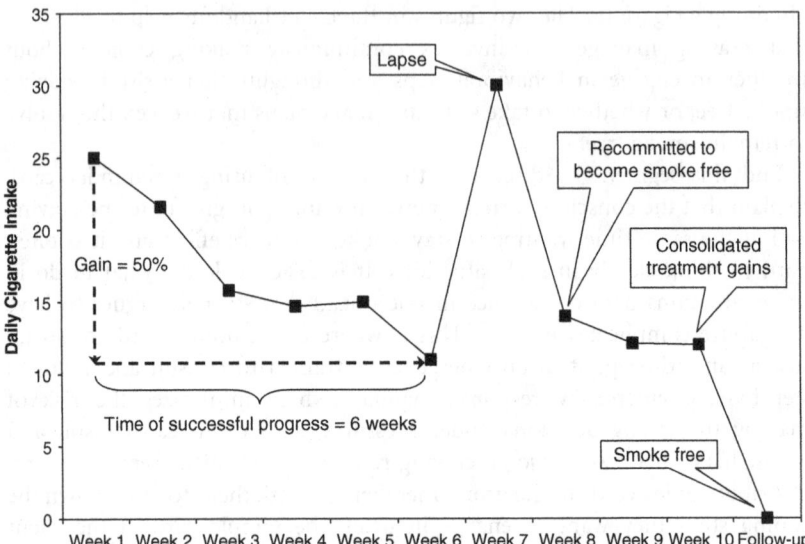

Figure 7.2 Example of using monitoring data to help clients to recover from a lapse.

steps provide a framework for discussing with that client what went wrong and how to do better the next time. In this context, the use of the weekly monitoring data is extremely effective.

Figure 7.2 illustrates how the monitoring data can be used to help clients to avoid getting discouraged after a lapse. The key is to focus on the gains made prior to the lapse, and to use that "hard evidence" as a benchmark for what the client is able to achieve. In this example, the client was able to reduce daily cigarette intake gradually from 25 to 12 cigarettes over the first six weeks of the program. Relative to her heavy smoking status at the beginning of the program, and relative to the nearly three decades of continuous smoking at that level prior to joining the group, this substantial and sustained reduction is a huge achievement. The graphic representation of successful gains is a powerful tool to help clients to realize that doing things differently leads to measurable and sustained change. In this case, after convincing the client to rejoin the group after her lapse episode (during which she had let it all go and smoked at an even higher level than prior to commencing the program), she was able to consolidate the changes achieved over the first half of the program. Although she did not manage to become smoke free by the end of the program, she quit in the week following the end of the program and was still smoke free at the one-month follow-up.

Tips for working with individuals

This module is introduced around the time that some of the group members have selected as their quit date. For most in the group, this tends to be around the fourth or fifth week into the program, but when working with an individual client the timing of quit day is unique to the personal circumstances of the client. It may come much earlier or later in the program, in which case it is best to cover the module on prevention and management of lapse or relapse around the time the individual is ready to quit.

Although the supportive group context is advantageous for helping clients to garner the strength and motivation to pick themselves up again after a relapse, the emphasis at this stage of the change process is for each client to take the responsibly for making the right choices and following through with their own personal change plan. In that sense, little adaptation is required when working with a single client.

To the extent that "counseling-type" activities may be useful for a particular client to learn how to cope better with emotionally stressful situations that could trigger a relapse, their incorporation into the treatment plan is much more straightforward for a single client. There is no need to gauge first the level of general acceptance of this particular treatment component within the group as a whole, or to tailor its delivery in such a way that it minimizes embarrassment in front of group members. Indeed, if significant emotional problems are undermining smoking cessation attempts, issues with confidentiality are easier to manage when working with individual clients than working in a group environment.

Similarly straightforward is the discussion of the worksheet used by clients to identify their personal high-risk situations. This discussion will be personalized with respect to the client's circumstances and, as only one client is involved, there is plenty of time in a session to complete these exercises within the session, rather than assigning the elaboration of the worksheet as a homework task.

When practicing refusal skills, this cannot be done in client pairs but is equally effective using role play within the client–therapist pair.

When introducing the material on managing setbacks to a single client, this can typically be achieved within the same session. Therefore, it is unlikely that the initial discussion of these materials needs to be distributed over two sessions, as is often necessary for group sessions given the greater diversity in themes that needs to be accommodated in the same amount of time. Whether or not all materials in this module are introduced in a single session is not critical, as these topics should be revisited anyway whenever they become relevant during treatment.

Tips (cont.)

Finally, as the *Client materials* make the occasional reference to a group context, individual clients can simply be advised to ignore those group references as all the guidelines covered in the materials are equally relevant in the individual treatment context.

CLIENT MATERIALS

1 How do I prevent a lapse?
2 What to do when a lapse occurs.

How do I prevent a lapse?

A **lapse** is a temporary setback or slip on the path to becoming smoke free. It refers to smoking one or a few cigarettes after at least 24 hours of abstinence followed by a resumption of the quit attempt. A **relapse** is the return to regular smoking, even if at a lower level than prior to the quit attempt. Lapses are common and typically occur shortly after becoming smoke free. A high proportion of smokers who lapse eventually relapse. However, a slip does not need to lead to a relapse! Knowing in what situations a lapse is most likely to occur for you personally, and being prepared to apply the right tools in those situations, will help you to prevent a lapse or relapse occurring. Lapse prevention is hard work and takes a lot of effort on your part. The group can help you every step along the way, but it is your responsibility to make a commitment to engaging in the **three key tasks of (re)lapse prevention**: (a) identify your personal high-risk situations, (b) practice and apply strategies to manage these situations, and (c) in the event of a lapse, control the outcome by choosing swift resumption of the quit attempt over return to regular smoking. The following table summarizes the most common situations where smokers attempting to quit are at high risk for experiencing a lapse, along with the strategies you can use to reduce that risk.

Table of high-risk situations and possible management strategies

High-risk situation	Management strategies
Negative emotional states (e.g., anxiety, frustration, anger, stress, depression)	• Apply stress management and problem-solving skills • Change unhelpful thoughts • Seek support
Arguments with partners, family, friends, or colleagues	• Use assertive (rather than passive or aggressive) communications
Social situations where smoking is taking place	• Minimize exposure to places and people associated with smoking • Apply smoking-refusal skills
Cravings and weakening of resolve	• Prepare and practice personal response plan • Consider using nicotine-replacement treatments or bupropion (Zyban) • Exercise • Use reminder cards to bolster motivation • Seek support (e.g., phone a "buddy") • Change unhelpful thoughts

High-risk situation	Management strategies
Withdrawal distress	• Consider using nicotine-replacement treatments or bupropion (Zyban) • Exercise • Remind yourself that withdrawal symptoms are temporary and will disappear within 10 days of quitting

Identify your own high-risk situations

To get a better understanding of what lapse prevention is about, think about the journey *From Smoke City to Fresh Hills* we talked about in the first group session. There are difficult and easy sections along the roads. The lapses are the difficult sections of the road. Signposts alert us to these upcoming dangers. The driver who is alert to these signposts and takes the necessary precautions avoids veering off into the difficult sections.

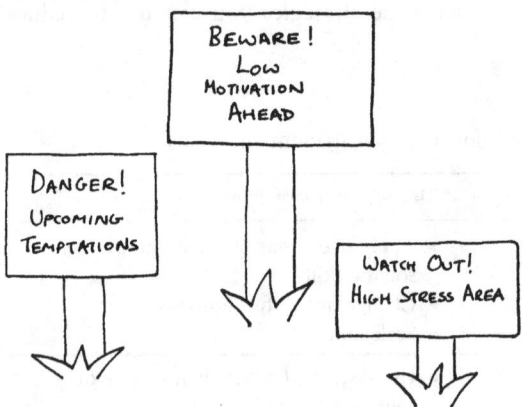

Relapse prevention requires you to be the conscientious driver and be on the lookout for signposts indicating potentially difficult situations. The sooner you spot the signs, the easier it is to anticipate what lies around the next bend. What situations are particularly difficult is not the same for all people. It is therefore a helpful first step if you identified for yourself what your personal high-risk situations are. Use the worksheet entitled *My personal high-risk situations worksheet* to list all the situations where you think you might be likely to have a lapse. List your high-risk situations in the left column, and indicate the level of risk (moderate, high, very high) for that

MY PERSONAL HIGH-RISK SITUATIONS WORKSHEET	
High-risk situations	**Risk level**
Negative emotional states	☐ NA
	☐ moderate ☐ high ☐ very high
	☐ moderate ☐ high ☐ very high
	☐ moderate ☐ high ☐ very high
	☐ moderate ☐ high ☐ very high
Arguments with partners, family, friends, or colleagues	☐ NA
	☐ moderate ☐ high ☐ very high
	☐ moderate ☐ high ☐ very high
	☐ moderate ☐ high ☐ very high
	☐ moderate ☐ high ☐ very high
Social situations where smoking is taking place	☐ NA
	☐ moderate ☐ high ☐ very high
	☐ moderate ☐ high ☐ very high
	☐ moderate ☐ high ☐ very high
	☐ moderate ☐ high ☐ very high
Cravings and/or weakening of resolve	☐ NA
	☐ moderate ☐ high ☐ very high
	☐ moderate ☐ high ☐ very high
	☐ moderate ☐ high ☐ very high
	☐ moderate ☐ high ☐ very high
Withdrawal distress	☐ NA
	☐ moderate ☐ high ☐ very high
	☐ moderate ☐ high ☐ very high
	☐ moderate ☐ high ☐ very high
	☐ moderate ☐ high ☐ very high
Other	
	☐ moderate ☐ high ☐ very high
	☐ moderate ☐ high ☐ very high
	☐ moderate ☐ high ☐ very high
	☐ moderate ☐ high ☐ very high

particular situation in the right column. To make it easier to think about potential situations, there are five sections, one for each of the most common categories of high-risk situations that smokers attempting to quit experience. If a section does not apply to you personally, leave that section blank and tick the box "NA" in the right column. For every situation you list, also tick the risk level in the right column. This can help you to become aware of some situations that may be more risky than others. For example, you may find stressful communications with an ex-partner about child-care arrangements to be a moderate risk for triggering a lapse, because you can usually keep contact brief and remove yourself from the situation quickly. In contrast, going fishing on a boat in close proximity with your smoking long-time friends may put you in a situation where the risk for a lapse is very high, because there is no opportunity to leave the situation should the temptation become overwhelming. There may also be situations that do not easily fit into one of the main categories. You can list those in the "Other" section on the worksheet.

Be prepared to manage high-risk situations

The first two sections in the high-risk situations worksheet are about emotionally stressful situations that can trigger a lapse. These situations could be ongoing and require so much of your daily coping strength that giving in to a lapse is easier than taking on the additional hard work of becoming smoke free. These emotional situations can also come up unexpectedly and overwhelm your still fragile status as a non-smoker at any given moment. There are specific strategies that are helpful in managing these general high-risk smoking triggers. These are covered in separate handouts entitled *Coping without smoking* and *How do thoughts affect smoking behaviors?* If you think those strategies would be useful for your personal circumstances, be sure to ask your group facilitator(s) to cover them in the group before your scheduled quit day.

The last three sections in the high-risk situations worksheet are about smoking-related cues (from within yourself or from your environment) that may trigger a lapse unless you apply strategies that help to take the edge of those tempting triggers. These strategies include (a) reducing exposure to places and people associated with smoking, (b) practicing smoking-refusal skills, and (c) managing cravings and withdrawal distress.

Reducing exposure to places and people associated with smoking

Traveling along the journey *From Smoke City to Fresh Hills*, you will inevitably come across many difficult situations. Sometimes, it will be best to take a detour – that is, avoid difficult situations altogether. While there will be situations that cannot be avoided entirely, it is best to avoid the more dangerous situations in the first few weeks of being smoke free, when the chance of a lapse is particularly high. In particular, socializing with friends who smoke in your presence, or sitting near or walking through smoking areas in public places are situations best avoided, at least for a while. Use your personal high-risk situations worksheet to highlight those situations where you want to minimize your exposure in the weeks after quitting.

Practicing smoking-refusal skills

While avoidance is an effective strategy, there are times when it is not possible. In such cases, you will need alternative coping skills to help you through these difficult situations without a lapse. One important skill is to be able to say "no" effectively when offered a cigarette. At some point in your endeavor to become and remain smoke free, it is likely that you will be offered a cigarette or even "bullied" into smoking by other smokers. It is good to know in advance what to do, and how to do it effectively, so that these social pressures to smoke will not trip you up should such occasions arise. This will be particularly important in the early period of being smoke free.

Smoking-refusal skills help you to respond to these situations with confidence and without making excuses. Before we look at specific smoking-refusal skills, let's look at different styles of refusal. Some styles are more effective than others. There are three general styles of refusal: passive, aggressive, and assertive.

- The *passive style* involves refusing offers in an apologetic manner. A passive response may be, "Sorry to put you out, but I'm afraid I've given up smoking. I am really sorry." Apologetic or timid responses often invite others to disregard the opinion of a passive responder, which, in turn, may lead to more persistent attempts to make you "join in" with the other smokers.
- The *aggressive style* is the opposite of the passive style. The aggressive individual conveys her or his opinion by attacking others. An aggressive response to an offer of a cigarette may be, "Look, I already told you a thousand times that I am now smoke free. Don't you listen? Just back off, okay? You can go right ahead and kill yourself with those fags." While this style is likely to make others yield to you and stop pestering you to smoke, this style leaves you feeling tense and agitated. This could backfire on you, as negative emotional states can often trigger the desire to smoke. It also could leave others feeling offended and they may then react in other unhelpful ways such as trying indirectly to sabotage your efforts to become smoke free.
- The *assertive style* sits between the passive and aggressive styles. Here, what you say and the manner in which you say it conveys your opinion of being offered a cigarette in a clear and direct way (unlike the passive style), yet it

still respects the opinion and choices of the person offering the cigarette (unlike the aggressive style). An assertive response may be, "No thanks. I'm a non-smoker now." This is the style that is most likely to achieve what you desire without offending others.

Now that we have clarified that an assertive refusal style is the most effective, let us review *how* one can be assertive when refusing cigarettes. Of course, if you already use an assertive style in such situations regularly, you can skip over these next few paragraphs. Being assertive when refusing a cigarette is not just about what you say but also about how you say it. Things to consider include making direct statements, being confident in your tone of voice, and using effective body language.

> *Use direct positive statements.* What you say is important in refusing a cigarette. Be direct. Do not "ummm" and "ahhh" as this conveys that you are not confident, which, in turn, may suggest that you are not fully committed to being a non-smoker. Also, do not attack the person offering you the cigarette by implying that she or he is inconsiderate and insensitive.

> *Use a confident tone of voice.* How you refuse a cigarette is just as important as what you say. Take the phrase, "No thank you. I'm a non-smoker now." Say it in a timid tone, an assertive tone, and an aggressive tone. Note the difference in these. Aim for an assertive tone where you are firm, calm, and unhesitating. Being loud and threatening may offend, and being shy and uncertain may prompt others to question when you say "no" whether you really mean it.

> *Use confident body language.* Body language, along with the tone of voice, affects how others view what you are saying. Even if a passive, an aggressive, and an assertive speaker all said the exact same thing, the body language would indicate they were conveying different messages. The passive person has the head drooped, the aggressive person adopts a threatening stance, while the assertive person looks the other person directly in the eyes in a non-threatening manner. Feeling uncertain about refusing cigarettes will show in your body language as you hunch or slouch, or avoid looking the other person in the eyes. This sends a message that you are not entirely convinced about your decision. Rather, make direct eye contact with the person offering a cigarette, and sit or stand up straight – these both create an air of confidence.

Putting it all together, there are *five simple strategies* to strengthen your smoking-refusal skills. When someone offers you a cigarette,

1 Look the person directly in the eyes
2 Speak calmly, and say "no" first, so that the person offering believes you mean it
3 Avoid excuses and vague answers: they make it harder to refuse and do not strengthen your resolve to be smoke free

4 Change the subject so that you do not get involved in a debate about smoking

5 If the person offering will not stop pestering you to have a cigarette, request that she or he stops asking.

Practice, practice, practice! It is far better to be able to say what you want well ahead of time than to be unprepared if the situation arises and look as though you are not committed to being smoke free. Vary what you say, your tone of voice, and how you stand in order to get a feel for what feels comfortable to you and what gets an assertive message across. One of the advantages of a smoking cessation group is that we can practice this in group, and you can get feedback from others in the group about how your refusal message comes across until you feel you get your point across easily and effectively.

Managing withdrawal distress

Many smokers report withdrawal symptoms following the cessation of smoking, but not everyone does, and for some they are only mildly distressing. Symptoms may include irritability, frustration, anger, restlessness, difficulty concentrating, light-headedness, disturbed sleep, anxiety, depressed mood, cravings for cigarettes, and increased appetite. Should you feel any of those symptoms, remember that they will be short lived! These symptoms are strongest only in the first week after smoking the last cigarette, and most will disappear within 10 days. Only urges to smoke and increased appetite may last for several months after becoming smoke free. Using nicotine-replacement products can help to take the edge off any withdrawal distress until it goes away on its own after a week or two.

Managing cravings

Many smokers experience cravings soon after they smoked their last cigarette. To manage these high-risk situations effectively, it is important that you understand how craving may or may not lead to a lapse. There are six simple points to remember:

- cravings can't make you smoke unless you choose to do so
- cravings are a signal for you to step up your resolve to not smoke
- even strong cravings can be resisted, if your resolve to engage in coping strategies is strong
- if you allow your resolve to remain smoke free to be weakened, even relatively mild cravings can trip you up and lead to a lapse
- all cravings, including strong cravings, will pass – most last only a few minutes
- until the craving passes, it is your job to engage in actions that strengthen your resolve to remain smoke free, rather than undermining it by taking steps that bring you closer to a lapse.

The figure below illustrates how an effective response to craving is all about making choices. The choices on the left side of the figure are those leading to smoking. Note that those are choices smokers normally do quite automatic-ally and without much thought or effort. That is why sometimes smokers feel as if they did not have much control over their craving. Yet, there are opportunities to put the brakes on at each step toward taking a puff from a lit cigarette. Better yet, the sooner you make the choice to take the steps on the right side of the figure after you become aware of an urge to smoke, the easier it will be to weather the urge without having a lapse.

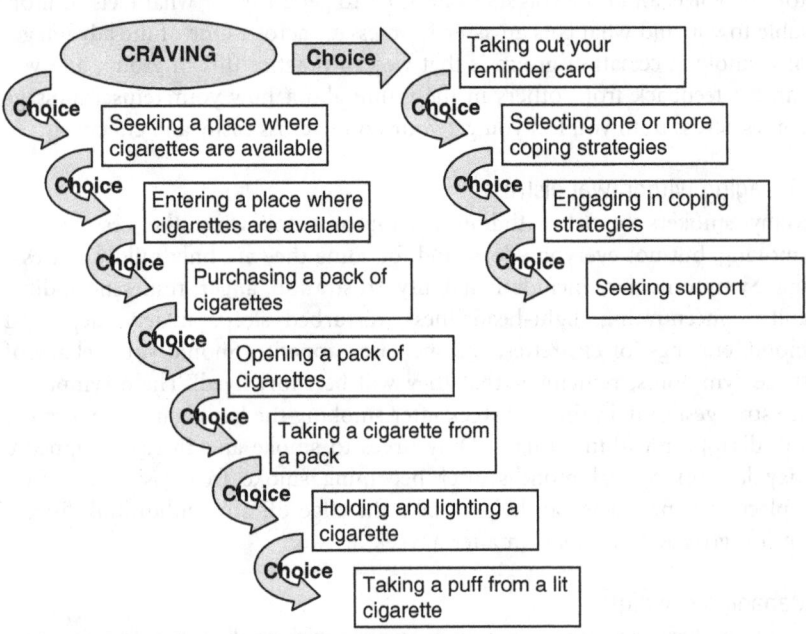

In addition to choosing to engage in *actions* that strengthen your resolve to remain smoke free rather than undermine it, it is important that you actively challenge any unhelpful *thoughts* that may pop into your head when you have a craving. Thoughts have a powerful influence on how we feel and what we do. If you allow unhelpful thoughts to occupy your mind unchallenged, your resolve to remain smoke free is weakened. Each time you catch yourself having unhelpful thoughts, replace them immediately with helpful thoughts. Some examples of unhelpful and helpful thoughts are given in the figure opposite.

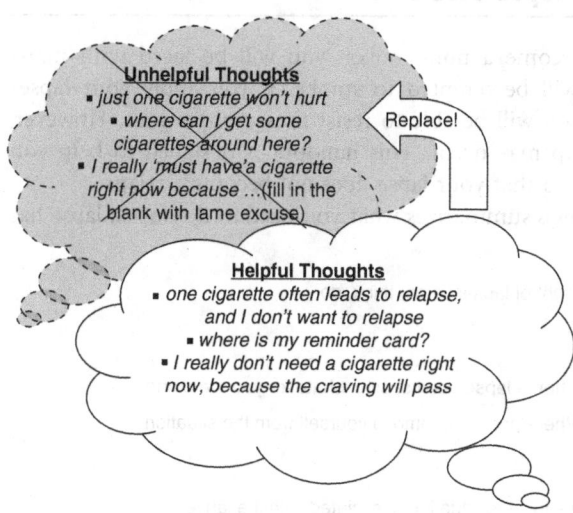

Remember that each craving you get through without having a cigarette is a positive step toward becoming a non-smoker for good. Each time you overcome the urge to have a cigarette, you will feel more able to resist the next craving. Over time, the cravings will get less and eventually disappear.

The reminder card is your personal "emergency" support system when you need to make a conscious effort to stay smoke free.

A sample reminder card

I can become smoke free and stay smoke free!
When I feel the urge to smoke… ▪ Get away from the situation ▪ Delay the urge to smoke – it will pass ▪ Drink water, sipping slowly ▪ Breathe deeply ▪ Do something else ▪ Look on back of card for helpful thoughts ▪ Call ___(Name)___ on ___(Number)___ ▪ Use nicotine gum
I want to be smoke free so that I can get more out of life!

What to do when a lapse occurs

On your journey to become a non-smoker, you will be faced with many situations where you will be tempted to smoke. If you apply your lapse-prevention strategies, you will be able to resist these temptations. However, in some instances, a slip may occur. This handout is designed to help you through such an event, so that your lapse does not become a relapse.

The *traffic light of lapses* summarizes what you need to do once a lapse has occurred.

The traffic light of lapses: stop, think, do

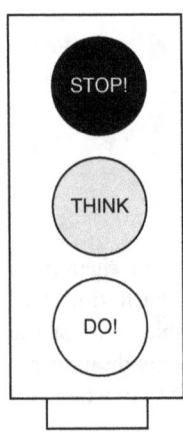

- When a lapse occurs, stop whatever you are doing
- Where possible, remove yourself from the situation

- Review the situation associated with the lapse
- Answer the question, "What triggers a lapse for me?

- Consult your reminder card
- Remain calm and challenge any unhelpful thoughts
- Renew your commitment to be smoke free

Review the situation associated with the lapse

In the event a lapse occurs, you are likely to experience feelings of guilt and blame (e.g., "I should have seen it coming"; "I am weak"). Put these aside for one moment and ask yourself matter of factly the following questions:
- What events led up to the slip?
- Were there any warning signals that preceded the lapse?
- What was the nature of the high-risk situation that triggered the slip (Where were you? Who were you with? How were you feeling?)

Asking yourself questions about the details of the situation (such as setting, time of day, presence or absence of others, mood at the time, and events that were occurring) will provide you with valuable information. The fact that a slip occurred tells you that something is happening that requires attending to.

Consult your reminder card

When you are upset and disappointed about a lapse, it can be hard to think straight. That's why we recommended that you make up your own personal reminder card. When one is distraught, it is easier to just follow an 'automatic' response plan that you worked out in advance, rather than trying to generate on-the-spot ways to get out of this dilemma. A lapse is a critical juncture in the road where your quit attempt has temporarily stalled. The reminder card is the jumper cable that will give you the spark needed to get your smoking cessation motor running again. The card should contain clear and easy-to-follow steps that you can use. Making the choice to follow the instructions on your reminder card immediately when a lapse presents a window of opportunity to keep the momentum of change going.

Remain calm and challenge any unhelpful thoughts

Above all, remain calm. The usual reaction to a lapse is one of guilt and self-blame. This reaction is only harmful if you give in to it and decide that you have blown your chance of being smoke free. Remember that one lapse does not mean that you are now a smoker. You can see your choices more clearly if you remain calm and allow your initial reaction to pass. Remind yourself that a lapse is not a failure – it is a wrong step, but more importantly, it is an opportunity to learn more about your high-risk situations. Examine your thoughts after a lapse. Are you having unhelpful thoughts that try to justify your lapse (e.g., "I really deserved this cigarette, I've had such a bad day, and I really needed this cigarette to unwind")? If you catch yourself thinking in this way, engage in more helpful thoughts (e.g., "After the bad day I've had I really did feel that I deserved a treat, but smoking was not the best option. What I wanted was to relax, and I used smoking to achieve that. But I can do other things that relax me. I don't have to smoke.")

Renew your commitment to be smoke free

Your motivation to maintain being smoke free is likely to waver following a lapse. You may say to yourself, "What's the use – I've blown it already." Again, this is a normal reaction and you can work against this self-defeating reaction by using the following strategies.

- Get out your *Motivational worksheet* and remind yourself why you decided to become smoke free in the first place.
- Think of the long-term benefits of becoming smoke free. Do you really want to give that up just because you've had a temporary setback?
- Importantly, look back at how far you had already come on your journey to become smoke free. Use your monitoring feedback sheets to reflect on the gains you have already made. Do you really believe that one slip cancels out all the progress you have made so far?
- Return to doing things differently to when you were a smoker. If you do things differently, the next time you are in a high-risk situation this past

lapse won't matter. What matters is that you take responsibility for renewing your efforts.

- You may need to take practical steps to undo any smoking-related steps you have taking during your lapse (e.g., getting rid of any remaining cigarettes immediately).
- Don't go it alone. Do not delay asking for help. Rejoin the smoking cessation program straightaway.

8

Staying smoke free III: coping without smoking

THERAPIST GUIDELINES

Aims

1 Explain the relationship between smoking and stress
2 Outline different types of strategy for coping with stress
3 Identify personal triggers for stress
4 Provide a structured approach to problem solving
5 Outline the keys to good time management
6 Explain the techniques for coping with physical stress.

This module is designed to help clients to cope with triggers for smoking. Negative emotions associated with daily hassles and stress represent a significant obstacle to being smoke free, and lapses are often preceded by increases in negative affect (Tsoh et al., 1997). The client materials for this module present a range of coping skills that center around the ability to manage negative emotions and stress. Not all of these strategies will be equally relevant to all clients, and some clients may not need extra coaching on coping skills as they already cope effectively on their own.

Techniques outlined in this module on stress management focus on behavioral and physical strategies, which include problem solving, time management, and strategies such as relaxation and basic self-care to assist in coping with physical stress. This module complements the module on prevention and management of lapses (in Chapter 7) and the module in Chapter 9, which focuses on cognitive strategies to assist in being smoke free.

The current module on coping without smoking, and the next one on helpful and unhelpful thoughts about smoking behaviors are meant to be administered flexibly in response to the group's predominant concerns and needs. For example, parts may be used earlier in the sequencing of modules if clients perceive smoking as an ideal and easy way to cope with ongoing daily hassles, and use that as an excuse to put off the task of setting a designated quit day. It may also be useful to challenge early in the program the myth that smokers will feel more relaxed when smoking than when they are not smoking.

Explain the relationship between smoking and stress

Begin this segment by asking clients to reflect on stressful situations where they have resorted to smoking as a way to help to deal with the stress. Clients typically express the belief that smoking helps to decrease stress. It is important in smoking cessation treatment to dispel myths about the perceived benefits of smoking, mainly the perception that smoking decreases stress (Health Development Agency, 2003). Point out to clients that nicotine is a stimulant and, therefore, should have the opposite effect! Highlight to clients that the reduction in stress is only a perception because smokers have a higher baseline level of stress than non-smokers and that smoking only serves to lower stress to a level that an average non-smoker would experience (Parrot, 1999). Follow this with a clear, reassuring statement that there are other simple strategies that are much more effective in reducing stress levels. Before reviewing those strategies, it will also be useful to discuss briefly with clients that not all stress is bad. You may want to use the graph in the client handout that relates different stress levels with performance to illustrate that a moderate level of stress can actually assist performance, and that the goal is to decrease excessive levels of stress – and maladaptive ways of coping with stress – rather than eliminating it altogether.

Outline different types of strategy for coping with stress

Introduce the two approaches for managing stress: the reactive and the preventative approaches (Schafer, 1992). Point out that many smokers use smoking as a *reactive* coping strategy for dealing with stress, and draw clients' attention to alternative strategies such as problem solving, time management, and relaxation. Then discuss the *preventative* approach to stress by introducing the concept of a baseline stress level. That is, the lower the baseline stress level, the less impact a particular stressful event will have. For smokers this means that decreasing the impact of a stressful event will decrease the need to smoke as a coping response. The concept of a baseline stress level is often easier for clients to grasp when it is visually represented. Draw two lines representing low and high baseline levels of stress, and then a third ("trigger") line above the high baseline line, representing the stress level that triggers the need to smoke. Then draw two "spikes" of a stressful situation of the same magnitude, one starting at the lower baseline, and the other starting at the higher baseline. Only the latter should cross the trigger line that prompts a desire to use smoking as a coping response. Explain to clients that the coping skills covered in their handout are a blend of preventative and reactive strategies, and while there is a place for both of these strategies, emphasize the importance of preventative ones.

Introduce the three categories for stress-management strategies that are mentioned in the client handout: behavioral, physical, and cognitive. State that in this module the focus is on behavioral and physical coping skills, and that cognitive strategies are covered in a different handout. Clients are probably most familiar with relaxation as an effective stress-management technique, but you can also discuss nutrition, exercise, and sleep as part of a preventative approach to stress management. Explain that the purpose of these strategies is to "set up good habits that will minimize the potential for stressful situations to occur."

Identify personal triggers for stress

Ask clients to reflect on the situations that typically trigger stress for them and encourage them to share this within the group. As you write these triggers down on a whiteboard or chart, group them into those categories found in the *Stress action plan* worksheet. It is not important that all categories in the worksheet are filled out. Some clients, for example, may not wish to talk about financial stressors. The aim here is simply to get a few personalized examples of triggers. Together with the examples listed in the sample stress action plan in the *Client materials*, these can be used to illustrate that there are effective coping strategies that can address each of these triggers. The benefit of this sharing exercise is twofold. First, it will stimulate and facilitate supportive group discussion, which is a key outcome as specified in training standards for smoking cessation groups (Health Development Agency, 2003). Second, by writing down these triggers of stress so that they are visible to group members, it will cue you to what strategies are best suited for addressing a group's particular needs, and thus provides guidance on what sections from this module are most relevant and what may be best to leave out. Following this group activity, tell clients that they can use the blank worksheet in their handout at home to draw up their individual *Stress action plan* by filling in the triggers in the left column, and their plan for doing something about it in the right column.

Provide a structured approach to problem solving

Begin this segment by discussing what problem solving is and is not. Highlight to clients that problem solving as a technique is not a stand-alone technique but rather draws on other coping strategies. To illustrate, for someone who wants to be smoke free it is not simply a matter of identifying the problem as "smoking" and the solution as "being smoke free;" in order to achieve being smoke free the person needs to draw on a range of techniques such as learning to cope with cravings, modifying unhelpful thoughts that maintain smoking behaviors, learning relaxation to help in managing stress, and so on. Thus, problem solving is a method to help to identify what the real issue is, and to identify the most suitable solutions. People often select a solution because it is the first one that comes to mind and it may be based more on emotion than on reason; problem solving aims to help in approaching difficulties in a more rational and structured manner.

Of course, for many smokers the first "solution" that comes to mind when faced with a stressful situation is to smoke a cigarette. Therefore, the next point to emphasize as a group facilitator is the need for clients to focus on solving the problem that leads to stress in the first place. That is, the problem that triggered the smoking will still be there after one has had a smoke – and it will not go away even after having a few more smokes. One way to get clients on board with learning problem-solving skills is to ask them what happens to their problem when they have finished smoking their cigarette. Is it still there, or has it magically disappeared? When challenged in this way, clients readily admit that smoking does not solve any of their problems. If anything, it *adds* many problems to their life. So the key to coping without smoking is to be aware and make use of alternative strategies to solving the problem at hand.

After this clarification of the role of problem-solving skills in smoking cessation, you can proceed to introducing the five practical problem-solving steps outlined in the client handout (D'Zurilla, 1988). How clients view the nature of problems is as important to successful problem solving as the application of problem-solving strategies, and so the first step to problem solving is to examine how clients typically approach their problems (i.e., the "A" in the ANSWER acronym used in the client handout). Excessively negative viewpoints about problems (e.g., taking it too personally, feeling hopeless about achieving a solution, engaging in self-blame) can get in the way of finding a viable solution. Stress that problems are part of everyday life and frame problems as learning experiences. After you have reviewed with clients the remaining four problem-solving steps as outlined in the client handout, you can illustrate the process of problem solving by working through one or two examples. You may wish to draw on those triggers for stress that clients identified in the earlier discussion of the *Stress action plan*.

Outline the keys to good time management

The aim of good time management is to minimize stress in the first instance by managing time effectively. Poor time management often contributes to the stress that prompts clients to smoke. As with problem-solving skills, it will vary from group to group to what extent issues of time management are relevant. Ask questions to prompt your clients to reflect on their time management (e.g., "Do you ever feel rushed for time?" "Do you find that you always have something to do?") and explore what impact it has on their desire to smoke.

A common observation is that having a cigarette break is viewed as the one chance that smokers get to escape from whatever is causing them stress. Ask your clients to reflect on how this increases the value of smoking to them? Does it serve to validate their right to smoke as a way of shutting the world out so that they can get some valuable time to themselves? Then ask them how it would be different if they were able to find time for themselves without using the smoking break as an excuse? Would their desire for a cigarette still be as strong?

The techniques outlined in the *Time management* client handout are easy to follow. It does not require much in-session time to explain them. They focus on realistic time estimation, prioritizing of tasks, planning tools, and avoiding roadblocks to effective time management such as perfectionism and procrastination (Antony & Swinson, 1998; Buehler, Griffin, & Ross, 1994; Ferrari, Johnson, & McCown, 1995). Clients who have indicated that time pressures contribute to their stress-related smoking can be encouraged to use some of those strategies from the client handout to learn to manage their time more effectively.

Explain techniques for coping with physical stress

Begin this segment by introducing to clients the fight or flight response, in particular highlighting that an increased breathing rate and an increased heart rate are part of the response. This will pave the way for the introduction of relaxation techniques designed to counter the stress response directly. Highlight the adaptive function of the fight or flight response, emphasizing that for the stressors we face nowadays fighting or fleeing are typically not appropriate coping strategies, and therefore, there is a need to find alternative ways to burn up the stress hormones circulating in our bodies.

Following the explanation of the stress response, introduce relaxation as a way of directly countering the stress response by slowing down breathing rate, decreasing heart rate, and so on (Davis, Eshelman, & McKay, 1995). Outline the options for relaxation: in the client handout we have covered relaxation through breathing, progressive muscle relaxation, and relaxation with imagery. It is recommended that you conduct at least one relaxation session with the group, which may or may not include imagery (see also Chapter 10 for examples of imagery exercises designed to help clients to practice goal-directed imagery to enhance the formation of a self-concept as a non-smoker).

Encourage clients to practice relaxation on a regular basis so that it will be easier to engage the technique when they are feeling stressed. Highlight that relaxation – in particular, controlled breathing – is a portable technique that clients can use in situations where they feel an urge to smoke in response to stress. Moreover, practicing relaxation regularly is effective as a preventative approach to stress management. In this context, reiterate the concept of lowering one's baseline stress levels as a means of lowering the impact of stressful events. Alas, while clients are probably seeking some magical strategies where prevention is concerned, it is the old combination of exercise, nutrition, sleep, and work/life balance that helps to minimize stress.

Typically, clients are already aware of the exercise, nutrition, sleep, and balance information but may experience difficulties in maintaining a preventative approach. The key to maintenance is that clients incorporate these changes into their daily routines. Some clients may find that too difficult, given that they are already dealing with the effort it takes to give up smoking. For other clients becoming smoke free is an important step in achieving overall better health and they are keen to take other steps that support that goal. This is where some problem-solving skills may come in handy. For example, if a client does not have time to exercise after work because of childcare commitments, he or she can use problem-solving strategies to identify solutions that would allow some time for exercise while making alternative arrangements for childcare. Similarly, if clients find it difficult to make time to relax, encourage them to review the time management strategies. In sum, the coping skills described in this module complement each other. They can go a long way in assisting clients to deal with the daily hassles and stress that all too often serve as triggers for smokers to lapse and waver in their resolve to become smoke free. Emphasize to clients that balance is particularly important in adopting a preventative approach to stress. If clients have used smoking as a crutch for coping, the prospect of coping without smoking is a daunting one. Without the confidence that there are effective alternatives, the value of smoking becomes overemphasized and it becomes easier for clients to justify smoking ("It's the only good thing that I have in my life right now"). Therefore, this *Coping without smoking* module offers clients step-by-step guidance on a range of effective alternative coping strategies. To the extent that clients effectively practice these strategies, the perceived value of smoking as a necessary coping tool will be diminished.

Tips for working with individuals

All of the coping strategies described in this module are readily applicable to the one-on-one context. Indeed, working individually with clients means that you can best tailor a combination of coping skills to match your client's circumstances.

You can personalize the sections of this chapter in the following ways.

- In the problem-solving section, use one of your client's examples to illustrate the process of problem solving and ask the client to work through another of his/her examples to illustrate to you that the principles have been grasped.
- In the time management section, you can spend more time focusing on your client's particular circumstances, assisting them to develop their own time management plan, and specifically addressing any roadblocks to effective time management that are relevant to this client.
- In the coping with physical stress section, you can tailor the breathing technique, progressive muscle relaxation technique, and relaxing imagery scene to what will fit best with your client. As part of the relaxation with imagery exercise, include an image of something that your client wants to do once s/he is smoke free. Creating positive imagery is important for motivating your client, and being able to tailor the image makes it more relevant for your client than a group-based image may be.

As a cautionary note, be mindful of becoming side-tracked when covering the coping skills module. Unlike the other modules in this book, which are more directly focused on smoking, the skills in this section can be applicable to other areas of a client's life and it is quite easy to end up addressing other issues that the client presents with. If this is the case, discuss with your client the need to remain focused on smoking cessation for now and, if appropriate, offer information about referral options.

CLIENT MATERIALS

1 Coping without smoking
2 Problem solving
3 Time management
4 Coping with physical stress.

Coping without smoking

One of the common triggers of smoking is negative feelings. Stress is one of those negative feelings that we deal with on a daily basis. While major stressors such as death, separation, divorce, and other significant changes are a source of stress, it is more often the daily hassles that can prompt a desire to smoke as a coping strategy. About 80% of smokers report smoking to be relaxing or pleasurable. However, because nicotine is a stimulant, it does not have a "real" relaxing effect. Rather, smoking seems relaxing because of psychological reasons – smokers generally have a higher baseline level of stress, and when they smoke this falls to a level similar to that of non-smokers.

Therefore, learning to cope without smoking will be an important tool to help you to stay on track to being smoke free.

Stress: it's not all bad news

We're all too familiar with the experience of stress arising from negative events such as arguments, managing our finances, interpersonal problems, or problems at work. This type of stress is easily recognized as it often reveals itself in the form of irritability and fatigue. However, positive events such as getting a promotion at work, giving a performance, or starting a new relationship can also produce stress.

The reality is that stress is not always bad; some stress can actually enhance our performance. In the figure, you can see that we tend to perform optimally

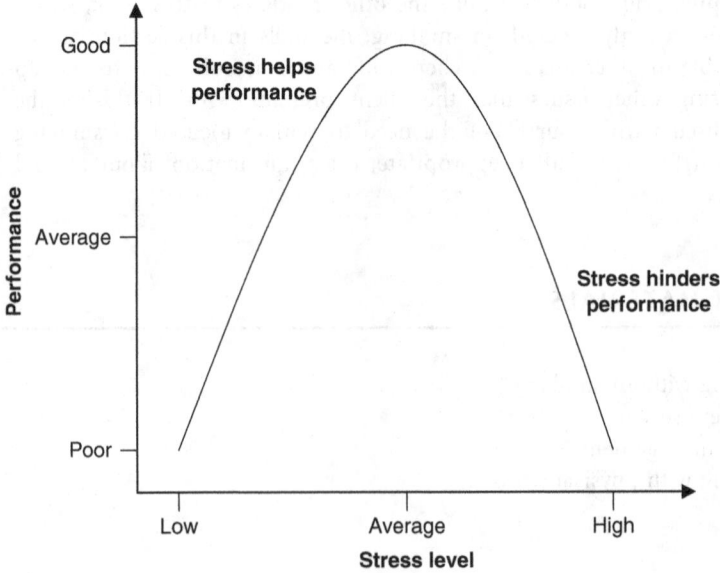

when there is some stress. Too much or too little stress, however, can impair our performance. The link between stress and performance can be observed in tasks that are physical in nature (e.g., some stress can lead us to run faster but too much competition can harm our performance) and also in tasks that require mental effort (e.g., some stress can help us to "cram" for an examination, but too much stress means that we are not able to think clearly).

Stress also becomes problematic when it is allowed to remain unmanaged for prolonged periods. Daily hassles such as minor conflicts with friends can build up to significant negative events such as loss of friendships, while problems with time management at work can build up to significant pressure in meeting deadlines, and in the extreme can lead to burnout. Stress can affect how we think, act, and feel. It can make us feel dissatisfied, decrease our enjoyment of activities, and make us inattentive to the needs of others.

Prolonged stress also has a real physical impact as it weakens our immune system and we become more susceptible to developing illnesses. Prolonged stress also contributes to high blood pressure, high cholesterol levels, and depression, which, in turn, contribute to the leading causes of death including heart disease and stroke. Moreover, smoking to cope with stress exposes you to additional risks such as emphysema, cancers, and other negative health effects.

Approaches to coping with stress

There are two approaches to coping with stress. One is to take a **reactive** approach, meaning that you deal with the symptoms of stress as they arise. Techniques such as relaxation, exercise, problem solving, and correcting negative self-talk that intensifies your negative emotions are ways of coping in response to stress that can replace the role of smoking.

Another way is to take a **preventative** approach, meaning you anticipate potential difficulties and take measures to decrease the likelihood of feeling stressed, or to decrease the intensity of your stress reaction. We all have a baseline level of stress and a "threshold" above which we experience symptoms of stress. By lowering our baseline level of stress, it will take more to tip us over the threshold. Preventative stress management strategies include maintaining a well-balanced lifestyle, time management, and learning not to overreact to situations.

Coping without smoking: what are our options?

For most people, a certain amount of stress is unavoidable, and as mentioned earlier, some stress can actually be beneficial for performance. By managing stress well, you can minimize any negative effects that it may have. Rather than coping with stress by smoking, there are better and healthier options you can choose to minimize stress. One easy way of looking at these strategies is to group them into behavioral (including social), physical, and cognitive strategies.

Behavioral strategies

Many daily events such as problems at work, conflict with friends or family members, deadlines, and financial problems can trigger stress. By applying effective behavioral strategies, you can manage these stressors better. Problem-solving skills (see the section titled *Problem solving*) are a good starting point to help you to identify what is the problem and what strategies may be suitable to solve it. Other behavioral strategies to help in managing stress include time management skills (see the section titled *Time management*), and assertiveness and communication skills (which are covered in a separate handout, *How do I prevent a lapse?*).

Physical strategies

You can use strategies such as breathing and relaxation (see *Coping with physical stress*) to help you to cope with the physical effects of stress. However, these are designed to *alleviate* stress, and a more proactive approach to managing high levels of stress is through good nutrition, healthy exercise habits, good sleeping habits, and regular rest and relaxation.

Cognitive strategies

Our self-talk and thoughts about an event can make us feel worse about stress than it actually is. Let's take an example of a meeting with a work colleague about budgets that involved some raised voices. One, less-helpful, form of self-talk could be "She's just out to slash my budget, it's like she's out to make life miserable for me and my department" – in which case stress levels and perceived threat would increase. Another, more helpful, form of self-talk could be "There are budget cuts all round so it's no surprise that my department is under scrutiny. Even though it is very unpleasant and I feel threatened, it's the bottom-line that she's concerned about, it's work and it's not personal" – in which case stress levels and perceived threat would be lessened.

Using more helpful thoughts and self-talk to decrease the intensity of negative stress reactions can go a long way to helping to manage stress and the stress-related desire to smoke. This technique can also be used powerfully to help in coping with cravings, lapses, and staying on the smoke free path. Hence, this is covered in greater detail in a separate handout (*How do thoughts affect smoking behavior?*).

Getting to know your triggers for stress

So far, we have looked at different options of coping without smoking. In order for you to gain the most out of the coping skills on offer, it will be helpful to identify those triggers that cause *you* stress. Of course, this will vary from person to person. This handout now gives a worksheet for your personal *Stress action plan* and an example of how to use it. By identifying your triggers for stress in various domains of your life, you are better able to tailor stress management techniques to your particular circumstances.

Stress action plan

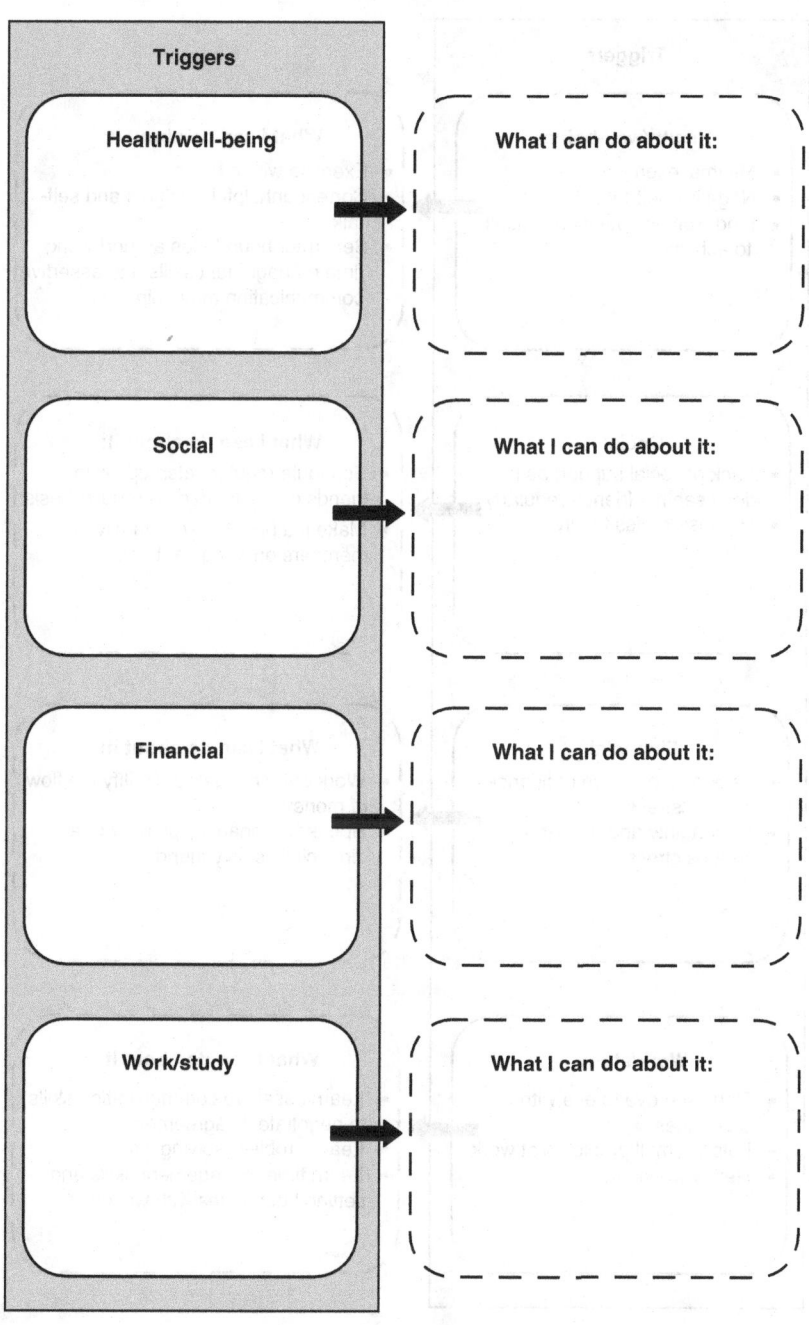

Triggers

Health/well-being → What I can do about it:

Social → What I can do about it:

Financial → What I can do about it:

Work/study → What I can do about it:

Stress action plan: an example

Triggers

Health/well-being

- Minimal exercise
- Negative self-talk
- Find work/life balance difficult to achieve

What I can do about it:

- Exercise with a friend
- Correct unhelpful thoughts and self-talk
- Set firmer boundaries around work; time management skills and assertive communication may help

Social

- Lack of social support as I don't see my friends regularly
- Homesick/miss family

What I can do about it:

- Schedule regular catch ups with friends or call them on a regular basis
- Make it a priority to call family members on a regular basis

Financial

- Lack of knowledge of finances creates stress
- Uncertainty about savings creates stress

What I can do about it:

- Work out a budget to identify the flow of money
- Speak to a financial planner or a financially savvy friend

Work/study

- Don't see eye to eye with colleagues
- Lots of small problems at work
- Heavy workload

What I can do about it:

- Learn assertive communication skills to negotiate disagreements
- Learn problem-solving skills
- Learn time management skills and setting boundaries with workload

Problem solving

Stress and other negative feelings often arise when we encounter problems in our lives, and negative feelings are a common trigger of smoking. Therefore, learning to solve the problems that trigger stress and negative feelings is a positive step towards becoming and remaining smoke free. Indeed, research has demonstrated that learning effective problem-solving skills significantly enhances smoking cessation rates.

So how do we go about problem solving? An easy way to remember the five steps of problem solving is to use the acronym **ANSWER**:

Examine your Approach to problems

Name the problem

Identify alternative Solutions

Weigh up alternative solutions

Execute and Review.

Step 1: Examine your approach to problems

Do you sometimes feel that problems are all your fault, that they will inevitably cause you significant difficulties, and that you are unsure if you have the skills to manage the problem? Is there a problem in your life that you wish you could handle better, if you just knew how to manage it more effectively? Are you prepared to put in the time and effort to change the problem or is it just something that you hope will fall into place?

The reality is that problems occur in everyone's lives. How we deal with them, and our belief in our ability to deal with them, are very important components of problem solving. For example, people may have very different approaches to getting a flat tyre.

Person 1   "Why me? I must be cursed. This is a disaster, I'll be late for all of my meetings and people will think that I'm irresponsible and incompetent. My manager will think negatively of me. How will I ever change this tyre? I've never learnt how to do so. People just don't bother to teach me things."

Person 2   "Oh no, a flat tyre. This is such bad timing – I've got several meetings back-to-back this morning. I'd better call to let them know that I'll be late. In the meantime, I'll call for roadside assistance first as they will take some time to come. This time I'll have to pay close attention to how they change it so that I won't be significantly delayed the next time my tyre blows."

Person 1 is someone who personalizes the problem and does not have the necessary skills to solve the problem. He focuses on the fact that he cannot change a tyre, and because he will be late for meetings, others will interpret it as him being irresponsible and incompetent. Rather than focusing on what he can do in that situation, he focuses on what he can't do, and ends up feeling helpless and hopeless. He may turn to smoking to relieve his stress.

Person 2 is someone who, while not having the knowledge to change a tyre, has a very different approach to solving the problem. While he may feel stressed, he also knows that focusing on the feeling will not produce results. Instead, he:

- identifies the major challenges arising from the flat tyre (managing meetings and changing a tyre)
- explores what he can and can't do to manage the challenges (call ahead to inform others that he is running late for meetings, calling for roadside assistance as he lacks the knowledge to change the flat tyre)
- learns from this situation so that he can engage in better problem solving next time (learning how to change a tyre).

By viewing problems as something that occurs to everyone, and treating a problem situation as an opportunity to learn a new way of coping, you are more likely to be motivated to work on addressing the problem.

Step 2: name the problem

Name the problem by clarifying what the problem is, based on facts rather than your interpretations. For example, looking at the thoughts that Person 1 had, let's examine what the facts were, and which thoughts were based on interpretation.

Why me? I must be cursed. This is a disaster

> *Fact:* Flat tyres occur to people everyday, they are not particular to one person
>
> *Interpretation:* Having a flat tyre it is not a disaster – it may be an inconvenience, but blowing things out of proportion can make the problem seem insurmountable

I'll be late for all of my meetings and people will think that I'm irresponsible and incompetent. My manager will think negatively of me

> *Fact:* You are very likely to run late for your meetings
>
> *Interpretation:* Thinking that others will think negatively of you is an assumption, not a fact; it is equally possible that colleagues will empathize with the bad luck and be supportive

How will I ever change this tyre? I've never learnt how to do so. People just don't bother to teach me things

> *Fact:* You don't have the knowledge to change a tyre and you've never learnt how to do so

Interpretation: It's unlikely that people don't bother to teach you things. It's likely that somewhere in your lifetime someone has taught you something, however small it may seem. So, while no one may have taught you how to change a tyre, they are likely to have taught you other things.

After looking at what the facts are, you can name the problem more clearly. In the above case, the problems to overcome are (a) the flat tyre, (b) running late for a series of meetings, and (c) managing the stressful reaction to the flat tyre.

There are two ways of coping with such challenges – to look at managing the problem or managing the emotion resulting from the problem. Problem-focused coping strategies are aimed at changing the problematic situation and can include time management, goal setting, and assertiveness training. Emotion-focused coping strategies focus on coping with your reactions to the situation in order to reduce stress and can include slow breathing, progressive muscle relaxation, and alternative self-talk (as part of changing unhelpful thoughts into more helpful ones).

Step 3: identify alternative solutions

Once you have clarified the problem, the next step is to identify a range of solutions to the problem. The idea behind this is that the more alternatives you come up with, the more likely that a viable solution will come up. As part of this process, put aside any judgements of how realistic or feasible each alternative is – getting caught up in why something won't work will hardly put you in the frame for finding out something that *will* work. If you get stuck, try combining alternative solutions or try expanding on a solution.

Step 4: weigh up alternative solutions

Now that you have a few solutions at hand, weigh up each solution to help you to decide which will be the best one to take on by looking at (a) the "pros and cons" of each solution, (b) how realistic the option is, (c) what barriers exist to the implementation of each solution, and (d) the effort and likelihood of expending the effort involved. Based on this, decide on the most feasible solution for you.

Step 5: execute and review solution

Once you have identified the best option, the next step is to execute it. In addition to barriers identified when weighing up alternative solutions, one "hidden" barrier may be your motivation to make the necessary changes. If this is the case, it may be wise to reconsider whether this option is a viable one, and whether you may be better off selecting another option (from Step 4).

Once you have executed a solution, review it in terms of how well it achieved the desired outcome. If the outcome was successful, then keep the solution in mind for use with similar situations in the future. If, however, the outcome was less than desirable, you have the option of returning to Step 3 (Identifying alternative solutions).

The example below applies these five steps of problem solving to a specific situation.

Problem	I have agreed to go out with friends who are smokers. I want to catch up with them but they've chosen an outdoor dining area where smoking is permitted, and I know that I will experience stronger cravings when I socialize with them. I'm feeling very stressed – I want to remain smoke free but I want to see my friends also
A: approach	There is a clash in what my friends want versus what I want. It's not an ideal situation, but I'll have to learn to manage by working out a compromise
N: name the problem	I want to see my friends. I want to remain smoke free. My friends want to go somewhere where I will be more likely to smoke
S: solutions	1 Refuse to go, telling my friends that I'm very disappointed that they didn't consider that I'm no longer smoking
	2 Go along with them
	3 Change my friend's booking to an indoor area where smoking is not permitted
	4 Call my friend and explain that I would like to go but will give it a miss because I may be tempted to smoke. Ask if changing the venue is an option and, if not, suggest catching up at a later date
W: weigh the solutions	1 Pro: My friends get to know how angry and disappointed I am with them Con: If it was a genuine mistake then I may jump the gun and offend them
	2 Pro: I keep the peace Con: I don't get what I want and I knowingly put myself at risk of temptation
	3 Pro: I get to socialize with my friends and minimize temptation to smoke Con: My friend may not be happy that I've changed his booking

4 Pro: I'm approaching this in a calm, rational manner, explaining my situation in case my friend doesn't remember that I'm trying to be smoke free. I'm raising the option of changing the venue, but if not, I have an alternative plan

Con: I can get a bit flustered with situations where I have to tell someone that I'm not happy. I'll need to learn how to speak my mind more assertively.

This is the most feasible option, but I will need to learn assertive communication skills

E, R: execute and review
Learned some assertive communication skills and plucked up the courage to talk to my friend. My friend was very apologetic as he forgot that I want to be smoke free and we discussed a suitable alternative venue. This option was successful in resolving the problem at hand.

Time management

Time pressure can often be a trigger for stress and, in turn, a trigger for smoking. Do you find that you are often running late, feel disorganized, can only react to tasks rather than plan them; find that even though you have free time that you don't get much accomplished; or find that you rush through things only to make simple mistakes? If you find yourself nodding in agreement with any of these statements, you may stand to benefit from improving your time management skills.

Strategies for time management

1 Be realistic about time management
2 Know how much time you *really* have
3 Prioritize and delegate where possible
4 Employ a vehicle for time management
5 Reward yourself and review regularly.

Be realistic about time management

Time management isn't a technique to help you fit as much into your life as possible. It isn't necessarily about making you work faster and, therefore, complete more. It's about helping you to streamline, and to be able to attend to those tasks that are critical for you to attend to.

As part of streamlining, it may be helpful to look at your overall aims in life to see how well your daily activities fit in achieving your overall aims. For example, if your aim is to spend more time with family and friends, then taking on more and more work and working at nights and on weekends is not going to help you to achieve your goal. Rather, setting limits on the amount of work that you take on may help you to achieve a better work–life balance. If you are a student and your studies are a priority, you may need to evaluate how much time for paid work and extracurricular activities you are engaging in.

Know how much time you really have

Feeling stressed from time pressures usually results from (a) underestimating how long tasks take and (b) overestimating how much available time you have.

> *Underestimating how long tasks take.* People often underestimate how long tasks take and do not leave sufficient time to complete tasks. How many times have you thought that you could give yourself 10 minutes to get to an appointment, not taking into account that 10 minutes means travel time only and does not include the time taken to leave where you currently are, get to your mode of transport, travel, find parking or wait for public transport, then get to the actual destination?

By underestimating how long tasks actually take, we put ourselves under unnecessary time pressure.

Overestimating how much available time you have. People often overestimate how much available time they have in any given day. That is, while it is easy to identify time spent at work, study, unpaid work, socializing, eating, and sleeping, people often overlook time spent on other tasks such as showering, grooming, preparing meals and washing up, doing the laundry, travelling time, ironing, vacuuming, answering the phone, having "down time" at the end of the day or on weekends, and so on. Failing to recognize that one also does all these other tasks can lead one to wonder where the time has gone and why it sometimes feels like one doesn't get much done in a day.

Quite often, underestimating how long tasks take and overestimating available time combine to create more time pressure and to cause more stress.

Prioritize and delegate where possible

Identify tasks that are priorities and tasks that can take a back seat for a while. Focus your energies on tasks that are priorities and delay tasks that are lower down the priority list for when you have completed these more important tasks.

Where possible, delegate tasks that do not necessarily require your particular knowledge or expertise. It may be as simple as getting someone else to set the dinner table, to check over a document, to write one part of a report, or to run their own errands where possible. Delegating can be difficult, particularly if you feel that only you can give the task the attention to detail that it requires. If this is the case, you can always check over the work if you wish, but in the meantime you have freed some time up for yourself to do another task on your "To Do" list. If perfectionism is a significant roadblock to delegating, check out the tips below (under *Roadblocks to effective time management*).

Employ a vehicle for time management

Optimal time management is achieved through good organization. So, get yourself a diary, whether paper or electronic, and use this to plan your days. Some people prefer using a timetable so that they know exactly what they are meant to be doing at each time of the day; others prefer the flexibility that To Do lists afford. Which strategy you use is entirely up to you.

Reward yourself and review regularly

Let's face it, time management may not be the most exciting activity in the world – very useful, yes, but not exactly exciting. Therefore, in order to keep yourself motivated to achieve those tasks that you set out to do, you can reward yourself. Sometimes, the sense of satisfaction from simply ticking things off the list is rewarding in itself. At other times, you may need an additional reward and this may take the form of some extra time off, or indulging in an activity that you enjoy.

Finally, review your progress on a regular basis. Your circumstances and routines change with seasons, holidays, different work schedules, illness, family problems, etc. This means that from time to time you need to review how well your time management strategies are working for you in light of changing commitments. Perhaps this will mean acknowledging that when things are stressful at home that your productivity at work may decrease a bit and to make the adjustment when setting out your timetable or To Do lists. Alternatively, it may mean temporarily scaling back on some social activities during a high workload period.

Roadblocks to effective time management

Among the roadblocks to managing your time are perfectionism, procrastination, and lack of motivation.

Perfectionism

Perfectionism can significantly interfere with your ability to manage time effectively. It can be difficult to overcome, particularly if you approach perfectionism as a badge of honor. If this is the case, it may be beneficial to examine how well perfectionism is serving you.

- Perfectionism can slow you down in the number of tasks you are able to complete. For instance, a report that you have written is likely to be sufficient for submission, yet perfectionism makes you constantly rework the report, making cosmetic changes that do not appreciably add to the report. This time could be better spent working down items from your To Do list.
- Perfectionism can make it difficult to delegate as you cannot trust others to do a proper job. This means that you take on every minute detail of a task, even if it is beyond your responsibility.
- As you take on extra tasks and take longer than expected on each of these tasks, you start to feel more stressed.

Decreasing perfectionism will involve making changes to your perfectionistic thinking. In perfectionistic thinking, "shoulds" and "musts" feature heavily ("I must do everything perfectly", "I should be able to handle everything, delegating is a sign that I'm weak and can't cope"), as does "all or nothing" thinking ("If I delegate one task, it means that I have failed completely", "If I relax my standards just one bit, it will completely fall in a heap"). If you find that perfectionistic thinking is an issue for you, refer to the handout *How do thoughts affect smoking behaviors?* to learn more about strategies on how to manage unhelpful thoughts and thinking styles.

Procrastination

Procrastination often arises because the prospect of completing a task generates some rather negative feelings.

- You may feel anxious or overwhelmed by the enormity of a task. Where this applies, it may be helpful to break down a task into smaller steps so that each step is far less overwhelming. Focusing on completing the one, smaller, step is likely to be more achievable than completing the larger overall task.
- You may sometimes feel bored at completing a task. One way to overcome this is to reward yourself after you have completed the task or parts of it, or do it concurrently with a more pleasurable task if the tasks are compatible (e.g., ironing while watching television).
- If feeling depressed when faced with a task is an issue, it may be helpful to examine why you feel that way about the task. Is it because you feel that you lack the necessary skills? If so, getting some assistance to help you to get on track may be useful. Is it because you feel that there is no point because you won't succeed? If this is the case, you may find it beneficial to look at changing unhelpful self-talk that derails your best efforts (refer to the handout *How do thoughts affect smoking behaviors?* for strategies on changing unhelpful self-talk).

Another reason why procrastination arises is because you may underestimate the urgency of the task and fail to prioritize this task. Quite often, people underestimate what exactly is involved in completing the task. One way to avoid this is to break down the task into the key steps that are required to achieving the overall goal, then to estimate how much time each step requires, and to see how it will fit in with your existing commitments and demands.

Lack of motivation

Why bother? You may sometimes feel that way about time management – why spend time managing time, when it could be better spent doing those things on your To Do list? Time management can be used to sharpen your effectiveness, direction, and your goals in order to decrease stress in your life. It can also help you to feel more in control of the events in your life, as well as help you to create work–life balance. While this technique may take some time and effort on your part initially, the benefits far outweigh the costs. If it helps you to stay smoke free, the benefits are huge!

Coping with physical stress

Our body's response to stressful situations – the fight or flight response – involves a series of changes within the body to prepare us either to fight or to run away from a threatening situation. When we perceive threat, hormones such as adrenaline (epinephrine), noradrenaline (norepinephrine), thyroxine, and glucocorticoids are released, which promote a series of changes within our body:

- increased breathing rate to help increase oxygen supply to the body
- increased heart rate to pump oxygen around the body
- increase in blood-clotting ability so that any blood loss through injury is minimized
- increased sweating to cool the body
- diversion of blood from extremities to those muscles essential for moving or fighting
- the mind becomes focused on escape.

The fight or flight response is an evolutionarily adaptive response and the hormones released prime us for physical action. While this may have been beneficial for our ancestors where dangerous situations concerned physical safety, our modern-day stressors require less of a physical response. Our stressors tend to include difficulties at work, problems in relationships, or stress associated with deadlines. In response to these modern-day stressors, our physical symptoms can seem unnecessary and very unpleasant. These unpleasant symptoms can include some or all of the following, for specific reasons.

- Feeling like you can't think straight: your mind is focused on escaping and not on other tasks at hand
- Shortness of breath/overbreathing and discomfort in chest: increased breathing rate; breathing quickly from the chest can result in chest discomfort
- Butterflies in the stomach: digestion is not essential to the fight or flight response, so blood is diverted away to muscles essential for a physical response
- Tingling in fingers and feet: blood gets diverted to those muscle groups vital for escaping/fighting; fine motor control is not necessary
- Pounding heart: increased heart rate
- Feeling faint: increased breathing rate, hyperventilation
- Sweating, body feels hot: cools the body so that it does not overheat.

Fighting or fleeing are ways of burning up the stress hormones generated when we perceive a situation to be threatening. As fighting or running away are not viable solutions to modern-day stressors, the stress hormones remain in our body. We need to find another way of burning up the stress hormones, or risk our immune systems being weakened and making us more susceptible to illness.

Techniques for coping with physical stress

For the techniques outlined below, we encourage you to use them in response to feeling stressed (e.g., relaxation when tension headaches interfere with your ability to concentrate on a task) and also in a preventative fashion to decrease overall stress levels (e.g., engaging in regular relaxation and exercise).

Relaxation

Relaxation helps to counter the fight or flight response in several ways, including decreasing breathing rate, decreasing heart rate, decreasing tension in the muscles, and slowing down brain-wave activity. Relaxation also has a widespread effect on the nervous system, meaning that it can help us to feel calmer overall.

Relaxation through breathing
Relaxing can be as simple as learning to breathe in a particular manner. When we start to feel stressed, our breathing becomes shallower and we breathe at a faster rate. By slowing down our breathing rate, we can bring about whole-body relaxation. The technique has the following components.

1 Breathe in and out *through your nose* only.
2 When you breathe in, make sure that you draw your breathe down to your abdomen, rather than breathing from your chest.
3 Select a relaxing breathing rate that suits you. The easiest is a six-second cycle where you breathe in over three seconds (in-two-three) and out over three seconds (out-two-three). Alternatively, if a six-second cycle feels too rapid, try for an eight-second cycle (in-two-three-four-out-two-three-four). Some clients prefer to hold their breath for a couple of seconds after inhaling before exhaling. It is ultimately up to you to select one that fits best for you.
4 As you breathe, you may wish to say the word "relax" when you breathe out. Another option is to visualize the tension leaving your lungs and then nostrils as you breathe out.
5 Attempt the breathing relaxation for at least five minutes; if you still feel stressed after this repeat it for another five minutes.

Breathing is a simple relaxation technique. It is also very portable, meaning that you can breathe in and out whenever you feel stressed without special equipment or others noticing what you are doing!

Progressive muscle relaxation

Our muscles can often tense up when we feel stressed, leading us to feel discomfort in our head, back, shoulders, chest, arms, and legs. Tension in our muscles can also lead us to feel tired. Learn to identify where you store your tension (e.g., in the face, the fists, shoulders and back).

In progressive muscle relaxation, the muscles of the body are relaxed in a progressive fashion, with the focus on all muscle groups. The manner in which relaxation is achieved is by tensing the muscles for approximately 10 seconds, then releasing the tension. Focus on the contrast between the tense feeling and relaxed feeling. A typically sequence for tensing and relaxing moves, as here, from hands to feet.

1 Fists (clench and release fists)
2 Forearms (tense and release forearms)
3 Upper arms (tense and release biceps)
4 Shoulders (bring shoulders up to your ears and tense, then bring shoulders down)
5 Head (raise your eyebrows, tense, then release)
6 Face (frown and purse lips, then release)
7 Neck (touch your chin to your chest, then lift chin back up)
8 Chest (tense chest muscles, then release)
9 Abdomen (tense stomach muscles, then release)
10 Buttocks (clench buttocks then release)
11 Thighs (tense thigh muscles, then release)
12 Calves (raise your toes toward your knees, then back down to normal position)
13 Feet (point your toes downwards towards your heels, then back up to normal position).

Relaxation with imagery

Your imagination can be a powerful tool in relaxation. One very effective imagery technique involves creating a relaxing place in your mind, a place that may exist in real-life or in your imagination. This is a place where you can see yourself feeling completely relaxed.

For imagery to be optimally effective, incorporate all of your senses – your sight, taste, sound, smell, and touch – where possible. To illustrate how to engage your senses to make the relaxation scene as vivid as possible, let's look at an example at the beach:

• walking on the beach with the warm, soft sand under your feet (touch)
• seeing the clear blue water and the fluffy white clouds in the sky (sight)
• taking in a deep breath and the scent of the ocean (smell)
• listening to the waves gently lapping against the shore (sound)
• lying under a tall, green palm tree (sight), feeling the warm sand under your body (touch)

- feeling the warm sun slowly melting away the tension in your body from head to toe, or feeling a cool breeze gradually blowing all of the tension out of your body (touch).

Imagery can also be a very useful tool in your quest to become and remain smoke free. You may wish to focus on the things you can do as a result of being smoke free, including swimming powerfully through the water as you are no longer short of breath, visualizing being able to taste food better, or visualizing climbing a hill and breathing in the fresh air at the top of the hill.

Contrasting images of yourself as a smoker and as a non-smoker is also another powerful imagery technique; you can focus on changes in your ability to breathe, changes in your ability to engage in physical activity, and changes in your image and appearance.

Relaxation: putting it all together

The relaxation techniques outlined above can be used in combination. Breathing, for example, complements the other relaxation techniques very well and can form the cornerstone of your relaxation exercises. A way of sequencing these techniques is to start off by engaging in breathing, move on to progressive muscle relaxation, then finish off by using the imagery technique. A few things are worth noting when attempting relaxation.

- Allow yourself time to relax, away from distraction. While relaxation via breathing can be used at any time, for the other techniques it will be beneficial for you to create time and free yourself from distractions to achieve optimal conditions for relaxation.
- Do not attempt relaxation exercises when trying to perform an activity requiring alertness (e.g., driving).
- Make sure that you are comfortable; this includes loosening any tight clothing.

Finally, relaxation isn't just for helping you to cope with particular stressful events. Using relaxation on a regular basis means that you work to decrease your overall stress levels.

Nutrition

What you eat impacts on your body's ability to counter stress. In particular, minimizing your intake of caffeine – found in coffee, tea, hot chocolate drinks, energy drinks, and chocolate – is advisable as caffeine is a stimulant. Adopt a commonsense diet that is high in fiber, rich in vitamins, and low in fat and salt. Limit your intake of refined sugar to avoid blood sugar-related mood swings, which may strain your body, and aim for a low-salt diet, as both stress and a high-salt diet can increase your blood pressure.

Exercise

Exercise is an extremely effective tool in managing stress in daily life and has been found to improve low mood. It decreases stress by allowing stress-induced adrenaline to be utilized by the body, and by releasing tension in muscles. Some forms of exercise can also help to alleviate "non-physical" stress by releasing frustration (e.g., boxing). Another benefit of exercise is that it helps to counter the modest weight gain sometimes associated with stopping nicotine intake.

Aim to engage in vigorous exercise (e.g., brisk walking, cycling, jogging) as this is the most beneficial for stress management. Although some exercise is better than none at all, aim for 30 minutes of vigorous exercise at least three times a week. Schedule in your exercise rather than fitting it in if there is time left in the day, and you are more likely to stick with it if you do an exercise that you enjoy.

Sleep

Sleep is vitally important to our well-being. Sleep deprivation or disturbance can lead to irritability, concentration difficulties, and memory difficulties, as well as emotional tension, and prolonged sleep deprivation or disturbance makes us more susceptible to illness. The amount of sleep that we need varies from person to person, so aim for an amount of sleep that leaves you feeling refreshed the next morning.

Some useful tips for sleeping include:

- Establish a routine whereby you go to sleep and wake up at set times each day. Start off by waking up at a set time each day, and if you feel sleepy resist the desire to nap as naps affect your sleep cycle. Gradually, your body will settle naturally into this routine.
- Avoid stimulants (including caffeine) for a few hours before sleeping.
- Try not to drink alcohol; while it may help you get to sleep sooner, it results in poorer quality of sleep.
- Ensure that the environment is conducive to a good night's sleep, including monitoring how noisy it is, how warm you are, and how much light is in the room.

9

Thoughts: how they affect smoking behaviors

THERAPIST GUIDELINES

Aims

1 Review the management of depressed clients within the group context
2 Explain the link between thoughts, feelings, and smoking
3 Introduce the four steps of modifying unhelpful thoughts.

This module complements the module in Chapter 8 and helps clients to develop skills in modifying unhelpful thoughts related to smoking. The role of thoughts in shaping smoking behaviors is critically important – particularly for clients who experience depression.

Managing depressed clients within the group context

The literature demonstrates an association between depression and smoking. Individuals with a history of major depression are more likely to smoke and be dependent on nicotine than non-depressed individuals, although the direction of this association is unclear. It may be the case that (a) depressed individuals self-medicate, (b) the withdrawal of nicotine elevates the risk of depression through the depletion of monoamine oxidase levels, (c) an interactive relationship exists between these two factors, or (d) there are common factors underpinning nicotine dependence and depression (Fergusson, Goodwin, & Horwood, 2003; Wilhelm et al., 2006).

Clients who experience low mood are likely to elevate the positive aspects of smoking and are less able to resist smoking when facing situations triggering negative affect or situations that are typically associated with their smoking habit (Hall et al., 1998; Tsoh & Hall, 2004). Framed in terms of the *Change cycle* (Chapter 6), current low mood – rather than a history of depression – is likely to keep a client in the pre-contemplation stage where they are less inclined to quit (Tsoh & Hall, 2004).

Studies show that cognitive–behavioral therapy has a beneficial impact on abstinence rates for individuals with depressed mood (Brown *et al.*, 2001; Haas *et al.*, 2004; Kahler *et al.*, 2002). The mechanism by which cognitive–behavioral therapy is thought to promote smoking cessation is by helping clients to manage the negative affect that triggers clients to smoke. That is, cognitive–behavioral therapy teaches clients alternative coping skills. While clients may still experience some negative affect, those undergoing cognitive–behavioral therapy are more likely to manage the affect without smoking (Hass *et al.*, 2004).

Based on the information gathered in the assessment interviews (Chapter 2), you should have a sense of whether depression is an issue facing clients in a particular group. If there are clients who talk about their depression in the group, encourage them to do so but be mindful of balancing the needs of these clients with those of other group members. In particular, if discussion becomes too personal and causes discomfort for other group members, refocus clients to talking specifically about how mood impacts on their cravings and smoking behaviors. Some clients may benefit from additional cognitive–behavioral therapy work for mood management independent of their participation in the smoking cessation group. In that case, consider providing clients with information about appropriate referral options.

For those group facilitators unfamiliar with cognitive–behavioral therapy, we have outlined the essential steps relevant for smoking cessation. Those interested in finding out more about cognitive therapy are encouraged to read the works of Aaron Beck and Judith Beck. Judith Beck's book *Cognitive Therapy: Basics and Beyond* succinctly outlines the components of cognitive therapy for those new to this therapy (Beck, 1995). Another useful and easy-to-digest guide on cognitive–behavioral therapy for mood disorders can be found in the *Mind over Mood* series, which contains a client workbook (*Mind over Mood: Change How you Feel by Changing the Way you Think*; Greenberger & Padesky, 1995) and a companion volume for the therapist (*Clinician's Guide to Mind over Mood*; Padesky & Greenberger, 1995).

Of course, unhelpful thoughts and negative thinking styles are also common among non-depressed people. The client materials in this module are designed to help clients to recognize unhelpful thoughts and thinking styles and use some cognitive restructuring strategies to transform unhelpful thoughts into more helpful ones. Begin by explaining the link between thoughts, feelings, and smoking.

The link between thoughts, feelings, and smoking

When explaining the link between thoughts, feelings, and smoking, focus on three categories of thoughts that are likely to arise for clients: (a) thoughts that prompt negative mood and a desire to smoke, (b) thoughts that justify smoking, and (c) thoughts in response to cravings and lapses. Begin by asking clients to review some examples of thoughts within each of these categories (see Worksheet 1 on smoking-related thoughts in the *Client materials*). Then ask clients to share their own smoking-related thoughts and write them on a whiteboard, grouping them into the above three categories.

Then, starting with the first category, ask clients to share recent examples of when they have smoked to alleviate negative mood. It does not matter whether the mood was anxiety, stress, or depression. Ask clients to reflect on what thoughts prompted the negative mood that led them to reach for a cigarette. As you do this, refer clients to Worksheet 2, the *Thought monitoring sheet,* and the example of its use in Worksheet 3, entitled *Thought monitoring sheet example.*

The next category of thoughts to elicit is thoughts that justify smoking. Sometimes, clients may feel reluctant to acknowledge the presence of these thoughts. If this is the case, reassure them that it is common that clients who want to quit smoking may still feel that smoking is justifiable at certain times. You can introduce this by asking clients to reflect on past attempts to quit, particularly on that split second where they have a fleeting thought – "I shouldn't be doing this" – in response to having a cigarette. The thoughts that follow the "I shouldn't" are of interest as those are the ones that justify the smoking behavior.

Thoughts that justify smoking typically elevate the positives of smoking ("I deserve it, there is nothing else going well in my life", "It's the only way I get to take a break from my stressful life"). However, a more subtle category of thoughts to be mindful of are those experienced by clients with anxiety/mood disorders, who may be reluctant to give up smoking out of concern that a relapse of symptoms may occur ("If I can't cope with it right now, how can I possibly cope when I'm not smoking?").

A third category of thoughts that we are interested in uncovering are those that clients have experienced in response to cravings or lapses. Ask them what thoughts typically pop into their heads when they experience cravings or smoke after vowing to give up. These are usually global, sweeping statements ("I'm so weak I can't even fight my cravings", "I'll never be able to give up", "No matter what I try, things will never change", "I'm back to square one"). Explore with clients what impact these types of statement have on subsequent motivation to be smoke free; it is likely that the perceived enormity of the task, and the perceived imminent failure at it, means that clients are less likely to attempt to quit again and have less confidence that they will be able to do so.

At the end of this activity, highlight again the power of unhelpful thoughts in keeping clients smoking. Then, introduce the concept of alternative, more helpful, thoughts to clients. This is the starting point to what in cognitive–behavioral therapy is called "cognitive restructuring." You could open this segment by posing the question, "So what would happen if, rather than thinking that having a craving meant that you were weak and will inevitably smoke, you are thinking that having a craving is normal and that you can do things to let it pass without lighting up? How different would you feel about wanting to light up?"

Introduction to the fours steps of modifying unhelpful thoughts

The four steps of modifying unhelpful thoughts are:
1 Becoming aware of unhelpful thoughts and so-called "core beliefs"
2 Identifying unhelpful thinking styles
3 Challenging unhelpful thoughts and core beliefs
4 Arriving at a more balanced thought.

Step 1: identifying unhelpful thoughts and core beliefs

Introduce the concept of core beliefs. Distinguish between automatic unhelpful thoughts (which are fleeting thoughts that occur automatically in response to a situation) and core beliefs (which are rigid, strongly held beliefs about ourselves and the world), using the analogy of an iceberg as outlined in the *Client materials* where the visible part of the iceberg is like the surface thoughts and the submerged part of the iceberg is the core belief. Core beliefs are harder to identify and change in comparison with unhelpful thoughts as they develop over our lifetime through direct and indirect messages that we hear.

To illustrate, you can use an example of someone who feels a need to be competent at everything and takes on many tasks, then feels stressed from too many demands and, therefore, smokes as a way of coping. The core belief here is that one needs to be competent at everything. This individual then interprets situations in relation to this unrealistic expectation of universal competence. The failure to live up to this ideal leads to feeling stressed, which, in turn, can trigger a desire to smoke. Encourage clients to explore the operation of their own unhelpful automatic thoughts and core beliefs by using the questions listed in the sample *Thought monitoring sheet* in the client materials. You can further illustrate the effective use of this self-questioning strategy with an example (also provided in the client materials) that shows a question and answer sequence uncovering the link from unhelpful thought to unhelpful core belief. Encourage clients to start using the blank monitoring sheet to monitor their smoking-related thoughts and feelings for a few days. As part of this, encourage clients to rate their mood and the degree of craving as it will cue them to those situations that are particularly challenging.

Some clients may have experienced difficulties unearthing smoking-related thoughts in the preceding activity. In order to bolster their self-efficacy for completing the monitoring homework, explain that this is because of the automatic nature of such thoughts, and that with practice this task will become much easier. A good analogy to use is that of driving a car. Driving is such a routine behavior that over time it becomes second nature and does not require much thought. In much the same way, smoking-related thoughts have become automatic so that they occur without one being aware of them. Learning to think consciously about them will be difficult at first, much like adjusting to driving on the other side of the road in a country with different traffic rules will initially require conscious effort, but with a bit of practice it can be done.

Step 2: identifying unhelpful thinking styles

Use worksheet 4, *Arriving at balanced thought(s)*, and the worked example of its use in Worksheet 5 (in *Client materials*), to introduce unhelpful thinking styles to clients as ways of thinking that maintain the unhelpful thoughts. Clients really take to this segment on unhelpful thinking styles and are able to identify easily which styles they tend to engage in. Your role as the therapist is to highlight how unhelpful thinking styles maintain smoking behaviors. The most pertinent of these are likely to be all-or-nothing thinking (they have either failed or succeeded), negative spotlight (focusing on past failed attempts rather than on progress such as the number of smoke-free days), and overgeneralizing (taking one lapse in one stressful situation to indicate that a return to smoking in *all* stressful situations is imminent).

Step 3: challenging unhelpful core beliefs and thinking

Cognitive work can be difficult to grasp, particularly for less cognitively minded clients, and it is better to go slower with teaching so that clients can digest the information at their own pace than to lose the engagement of clients through frustration. Step 3 could, therefore, be presented in a subsequent session to allow clients first an opportunity to engage in thought monitoring between sessions.

Introduce cognitive restructuring as a way of "replacing unhelpful thoughts with more helpful ones" and "tuning our thoughts" so that any resulting negative mood is less intense. Next, engage clients in cognitive restructuring by asking them to be thought detectives. Their role is to find evidence for the unhelpful thought, and evidence against the unhelpful thought. Of course, clients usually have plenty of evidence for the unhelpful thought up their sleeves. Your role in this instance is to test the generalizability of the evidence. For example, a client may joke that he has tried to give up smoking four times but obviously failed because he is in the group now! He believes that this shows that he is weak and he is likely to fail again this time. In this instance, you can acknowledge that he may have succumbed to smoking on four occasions, but ask him if at any point during those four attempts, he was ever offered a cigarette and was able to refuse it. If he was able to, this is evidence *against* the unhelpful thought that "I am weak; I'll never be able to be smoke free." Clients usually need some coaching in coming up with evidence against their unhelpful thoughts.

Throughout the process of engaging clients in cognitive restructuring, encourage them to conduct mini-experiments to test the veracity of their thoughts and beliefs (this is the behavioral component of cognitive–behavioral therapy). If they have the belief that delaying smoking a cigarette makes it impossible to concentrate and get their work done, get them to test it out by locking away their cigarettes for a couple of hours and use an alternative coping skill (Chapter 8). After completing the experiment, get clients to reflect on how true the initial belief is. A single experiment is unlikely to turn around a belief entirely; rather our aim is to open up the possibility of an alternative belief. Thus, if the experiment weakens the strength of the belief, this alone is an achievement. Successful behavioral experiments can then contribute evidence against the unhelpful beliefs.

Step 4: arriving at a more balanced thought

Once the validity of the unhelpful thought or belief has been undermined by contrary evidence, the final step is to generate a balanced thought, taking into account the evidence both for and against the unhelpful thought. It is important that you mention that the thought needs to be balanced, *not* positive. Distinguish between the two by stating that the balanced thoughts take into account that there have been past failures, rather than only looking at the bright side; in doing so, it enhances the believability of the thought. Using the above example of the client having failed on four past attempts to quit smoking, a balanced thought could be "While my last four attempts to be smoke free have not been successful, I have successfully refused cigarettes in the past, and by coming along to the group I will learn different coping skills to help me to manage without resorting to smoking; this means I have what it takes to become smoke free."

Some clients may baulk at the amount of effort involved in recording their thoughts, gathering evidence, and constructing balanced thoughts. As the therapist, acknowledge that it may be difficult at first to master but will get easier with practice to the point where the process of identifying unhelpful thoughts and challenging them occurs without the need to write them down. Again, using the analogy of driving a car while adjusting to unfamiliar traffic rules will be helpful here.

Finally, always praise your clients when they complete their between-session work and engage in cognitive restructuring activities. It is a tricky concept for clients to grasp, so it will require patience on the part of the therapist.

Tips for working with individuals

All the activities described in this module can be used when working with an individual client. Individual treatment may be the preferred option for some depressed clients as their needs may not be adequately met in the group context. Their negative thinking styles are more pervasive, and the strategies described here for dealing with unhelpful thoughts are geared toward the specific aim of aiding smoking cessation rather than alleviating mood disorders. The latter is likely to require specialist care and can be better addressed with a treatment plan tailored to the individual and that integrates smoking cessation strategies with the more primary mood management intervention. At the time of the assessment interview, it should be determined if a client with mood disorders is appropriate for the group or would benefit more from individual treatment.

When working with an individual client, bear in mind that clients will differ in their ability to understand the concepts and techniques of cognitive interventions. Some clients will grasp these techniques quickly, while others will require more practice, and yet others may feel more comfortable with the behavioral rather than cognitive strategies. Those slow to grasp these concepts can benefit from the greater personal attention in one-on-one treatment, whereas for those responding better to behavioral interventions, the materials in this module may be less relevant.

CLIENT MATERIALS

1 How do thoughts affect smoking behavior?

How do thoughts affect smoking behavior?

It may not seem like an obvious link, but thoughts play an important role in smoking behavior. Understanding how you *think* will help you in becoming smoke free in the following ways:

- understanding thoughts that prompt a desire to smoke
- understanding those thoughts that lead us to smoke in spite of wanting to become smoke free – we call these *thoughts that justify smoking behaviors*
- examining the way you think will help you to cope with cravings and lapses.

Thoughts that prompt the desire to smoke

One reason why smokers light up is because of habit without giving it much thought. At other times, negative feelings can trigger a desire to smoke. Feeling anxious, feeling depressed, feeling stressed – these are all emotions that can trigger the use of smoking as a coping strategy. In order to eliminate the need to light up as a coping tool for negative emotions, one can change the source of the problem (how one views or thinks about the situation). For example, if someone feels stressed at work, one can look at unhelpful thoughts that drive the negative feelings that trigger a desire to smoke. So, one can work on decreasing the perceived need to smoke by modifying the thought "It's all too much, I can't handle all this work" with "There's so much to do here, but I know that if I start to panic I'm more likely to resort to smoking. If I use the time management and goal-setting strategies I will feel less overwhelmed and more in control of the situation. I can get through this without using smoking as a crutch."

Thoughts that justify smoking behaviors

Once a craving occurs, there are two possible paths. One is to resist the craving and maintain on the smoke-free path; the other is to smoke. Certainly, resisting cravings can be very difficult, as you probably already know. What may seem less obvious is the internal conflict that occurs even if a choice to smoke is made; on the one hand, you have joined this program to help you become smoke free, on the other hand you are experiencing really strong cravings that you feel powerless against. Remember – you can want to avoid smoking *and* want to approach smoking both at the same time.

What we are interested in here are those thoughts that can tip you over into smoking. These may include overemphasizing the positive qualities of smoking (e.g., "There's nothing else positive in my life right now") or justifying your right to smoke (e.g., "After the day I've had, I really deserve a cigarette!", "I couldn't help myself, the situation was just too tempting").

By uncovering these thoughts and being aware of them, you stand a better chance of addressing them so that you can remain on the smoke free path.

Thoughts in response to cravings and lapses

The period following cravings and lapses is a high-risk one – one often feels less resilient, has less belief in one's ability to be smoke free, and is more likely to engage in self-blame. These all contribute to feeling worse about oneself, which, in turn, may prompt one to light up again. By examining the way *you* think in the face of strong cravings or lapses you help to put yourself back on track to becoming smoke free, and decrease the risk of falling into relapse. We will look at challenging unhelpful thoughts if such a situation arises, and replacing them with more helpful thoughts.

The figure below ties together some examples of thoughts that may affect smoking behavior. The corresponding Worksheet 1 at the end of this handout is for you to write down the most common thoughts that you personally experience in relation to cravings, justifying smoking, and lapses. Keep this worksheet handy so that you can remind yourself of unhelpful thoughts that you experience on a regular basis.

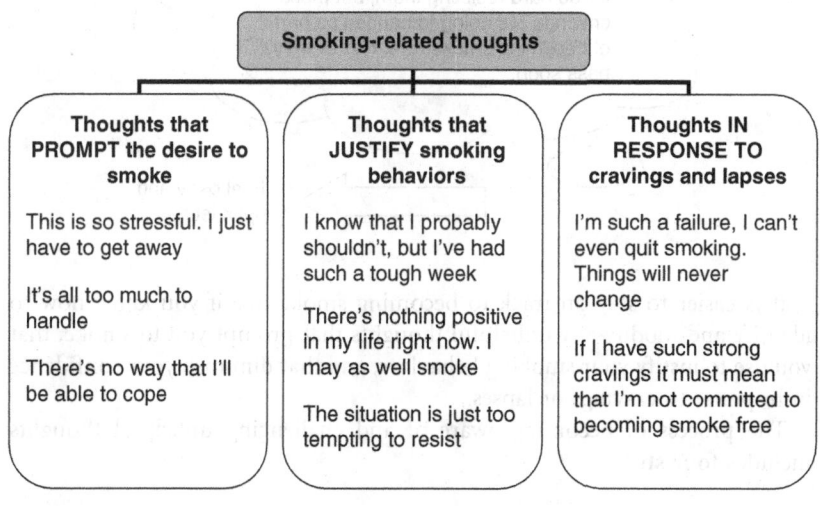

Identifying and correcting unhelpful thoughts

How we think about an event has a powerful impact on how we feel. The same event can result in very different emotions depending on our *interpretation* of the event, or rather, what we say to ourselves. For instance, many on the journey to becoming smoke free will experience cravings from time to time. How you interpret the experience of having cravings can make you feel either guilty and hopeless or "okay," depending on what you say to yourself.

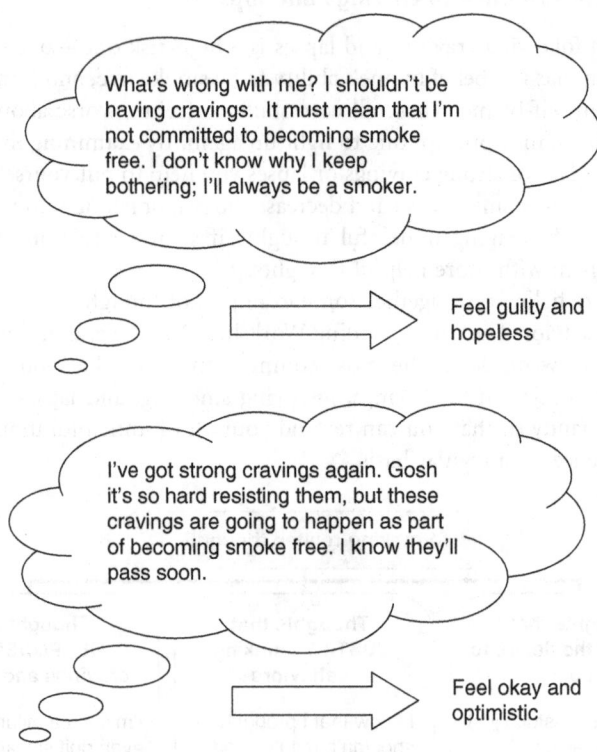

It is easier to stay on track to becoming smoke free if you know how to identify and modify any unhelpful thoughts that prompt you to smoke, that you use to justify your smoking behaviors, and that diminish your confidence in response to cravings or lapses.

The process of becoming aware of and challenging unhelpful thoughts includes **four steps**.

Step 1: becoming aware of unhelpful thoughts and core beliefs
Identifying unhelpful thoughts can be tricky at times. Quite often, all that we experience is the situation and then a feeling – the thought underlying the feeling is often not easily accessible. One way to help to catch unhelpful thoughts is to record them when your mood changes for the worse. An example of this is provided in Worksheet 3 at the end of this handout together with Worksheet 2, which is blank for you to use.

Do you need to record every single event just in case you experience an unhelpful thought? In short, the answer is no. The best indicator that an unhelpful thought is occurring is your mood – feeling guilty, stressed, anxious, or depressed are all signs that there may be unhelpful thoughts working against you. As a general guide, it is easier to fill in the situation and feeling columns – the thought column may be a bit trickier. To help you to identify those unhelpful thoughts, ask yourself the following questions:

- "What was I thinking right before I felt this way?"
- "What is the 'worst case scenario' that may occur?"

Unhelpful thoughts are like the tip of the iceberg. It's good that we can spot them, but we want to get to the part that is hidden underwater – the core beliefs. Core beliefs are strongly held beliefs about ourselves and about the world, and are harder to identify and shift than the surface unhelpful thoughts. They develop over the course of our lifetime through messages we receive from others as well as our experiences. To elicit core beliefs, ask yourself the following questions once you have uncovered unhelpful thoughts:

- "If this thought is true, what's so bad about it?"
- "What does this say about me and my abilities?"
- "What does it say about other people?"
- "What does it say about how the world works?"
- "What does it say about the future?"

An example of this may be:

> *Unhelpful thought*: "I should have known that going to a bar where others would offer me a cigarette would put me in a difficult position. I'm stupid and irresponsible."
>
> *Ask*: "If this thought is true, what's so bad about it?"
>
> *Answer*: "Well, the fact that I hesitated when someone offered me a cigarette – that I even paused before saying no –"
>
> *Ask*: "What does this say about me and my abilities?"
>
> *Answer*: "It means that I'm not committed to being smoke free."
>
> *Ask*: "So what would that mean for the future?"
>
> *Answer*: "Well, it would mean that I'll always have to keep an eye out for vulnerable situations; I can't ever let my guard down or I will fail. I'll always struggle between wanting to approach and wanting to avoid cigarettes."
>
> *Ask*: "If this thought is true, what's so bad about it?"
>
> *Unhelpful core belief surfaces*: "It means that I'm weak and will always be weak."

Initially, you may find it a bit difficult to elicit the unhelpful thoughts and core beliefs. With practice, you will be able to ask yourself questions so that you can move easily from unhelpful thoughts to core beliefs. You may wonder why unhelpful thoughts are so difficult to uncover. This is because they are automatic and occur without you willing them on, in much the same way that we become so well practiced at driving a car that it becomes second nature to us. Suddenly to be put in a position where we drive on the other side of the road will take some adjustment at first, but with practice a new automatic pattern can be established.

Step 2: identifying unhelpful thinking styles

Over time and with lots of practice, we may even develop unhelpful thinking *styles*, which are ways of seeing the world that maintain unhelpful thoughts. In the textbox below are some examples of unhelpful thinking styles. If you notice that you tend to have quite a few unhelpful thoughts, try to identify if one of those unhelpful thinking styles is present.

Unhelpful Thinking Styles

Negative spotlight
This refers to focusing on the negatives and ignoring the positives. This is particularly applicable to situations in which a lapse has occurred if one focuses on the immediate failure and neglects all prior successes including the learning and progress that have taken place. Suddenly, in response to one single slip up, all past accomplishments become worthless.

Catastrophizing
Catastrophizing refers to a tendency to assume the worst outcome. If a lapse occurs, one focuses on the worst-case scenario of inevitable chain smoking for the rest of one's days followed by death from smoking. Dramatic, isn't it?

All-or-nothing thinking
In all-or-nothing thinking, there are only extremes. It's either good or bad, black or white, all or nothing. Thus, lapses see you move from the "bright side" of total abstinence to the "dark side" of total relapse, with no middle ground. This style of thinking then leads you to believe "what's the point" and consequently you start smoking again.

Jumping to conclusions
In jumping to conclusions, we draw conclusions without facts to support them. This includes predictive thinking where you believe things will inevitably turn out badly, for example if you experience cravings you expect that you are headed for a lapse. It may also include mind reading, where we feel others judge us negatively without real proof. For example, we may think that others perceive us as being weak because we have tried to become smoke free on several occasions without success.

Emotional reasoning
Emotional reasoning refers to a tendency to ignore facts and instead to believe that the way we feel about a situation reflects the actual situation. For example, we may believe that because we *feel* like a failure that we *are* incompetent. With respect to becoming smoke free, just because you may feel disappointed that others in the group progress at a faster rate than you do at setting a quit day or counting their smoke-free days/weeks, this does *not* mean that you can't achieve the same smoke-free status a little later.

"Shoulds" and "musts"
Believing that people and the world *should* and *must* work in particular ways creates unrealistically high expectations that are unlikely to be met. When these expectations are not met, negative feelings arise. For example, believing that you should never ever feel a desire to smoke now that you have made up your mind to become smoke free sets up an unrealistic expectation as experiencing cravings are normal. However, feeling like a failure for having experienced a craving can lead to feeling guilty and pessimistic about your likelihood of success.

Step 3: challenging unhelpful thoughts and core beliefs

Now that you have some idea of how to identify unhelpful thoughts, core beliefs, and unhelpful thinking styles, you can start to challenge those thoughts that lead you to feel negative about yourself and may lead you to want to smoke. We will focus on challenging the core beliefs as these are at the root of it all. The best way to counter core beliefs is to examine the factual evidence both for and against that belief. That is, what is really the state of things and not what it feels like to you as emotional reasoning would dictate.

At first, it will be easy to find evidence *for* the unhelpful core belief and more difficult to find evidence *against* it. Years of practice have made it easy to have unhelpful thoughts, and making adjustments can be difficult. To help you to get started, some questions you can ask yourself include:

- "If my best friend was in the same situation, what would I say to him/her?"
- "How differently would I see this if I wasn't feeling stressed/guilty/depressed?"
- "Is there anything, however small, that contradicts my thought, but that I am discounting because I think it is trivial?"
- "Has a similar situation occurred in the past? How well was I able to cope? How well was I able to manage the unpleasant feelings that arose?"

Step 4: arriving at a more balanced thought

Now that you have found evidence for and against your unhelpful core belief, you will use the evidence to arrive at a more balanced thought. Balanced thoughts are often confused with positive statements, but the critical difference is that balanced thoughts are realistic and take into account evidence for and against the unhelpful core belief, rather than only focusing on what is positive. The reason for this is that the alternative thought needs to be believable otherwise it will not be effective, and only being positive is not likely to be believable when you are feeling negative about yourself, or have doubts about your resolve to become smoke free. An example of arriving at a balanced thought, after examining the evidence for and against the unhelpful core belief, is shown in Worksheet 5 at the end of this handout.

In the example, the balanced statement acknowledges that there has been a moment of vulnerability, but it also acknowledges that the vulnerability will pass and that a concrete plan can be implemented to prevent vulnerability in the future. Importantly, the balanced thought decreases the intensity of anger and hopelessness relative to the initial automatic thought and core belief. Use the blank Worksheet 4, photocopying as many as you need to, to help you to identify and challenge unhelpful thoughts, and then to arrive at a more balanced thought.

Putting it all together: challenging unhelpful core beliefs related to smoking

You now know the steps to challenging unhelpful beliefs. While these steps can be used for any situation where unhelpful beliefs can get the better of you, let's see how they can be put to use with smoking behaviors.

Cravings

Experiencing cravings can often lead us to think that we are not committed to being smoke free or that we are weak. This is a sign that there are *shoulds* and *musts* working against us. Perhaps you feel that you should not be experiencing cravings at all given that you have vowed to become smoke free. Perhaps you may also engage in overgeneralization and predictive thinking and believe that a lapse is inevitable. You may also have a tendency to shine the negative spotlight on cravings and to ignore all those times when you have not experienced cravings, or have successfully resisted cravings.

A balanced thought in response to cravings would be to remind ourselves that cravings are normal and related to the effects of nicotine withdrawal rather than to our commitment to be smoke free. Experiencing a craving does not mean that we will automatically revert to smoking; we are not at the mercy of cravings and have the choice and power whether to act on it or not (see the separate handout *How do I prevent a lapse?* on making helpful choices in the management of craving).

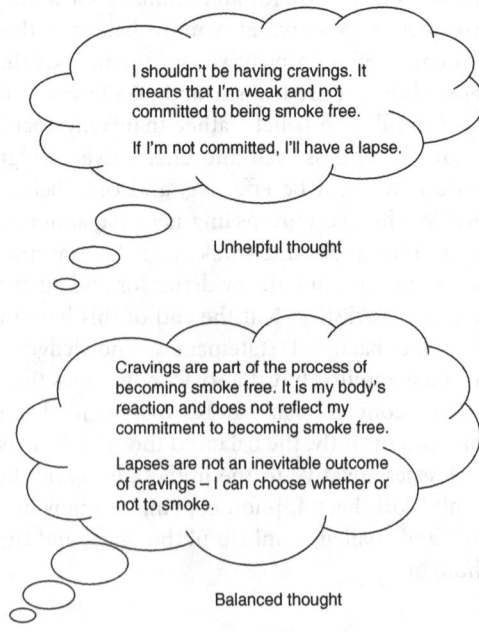

I shouldn't be having cravings. It means that I'm weak and not committed to being smoke free.

If I'm not committed, I'll have a lapse.

Unhelpful thought

Cravings are part of the process of becoming smoke free. It is my body's reaction and does not reflect my commitment to becoming smoke free.

Lapses are not an inevitable outcome of cravings – I can choose whether or not to smoke.

Balanced thought

Justifying smoking behaviors

Challenging thoughts that justify smoking behaviors are a bit different to the other types of thoughts that we have examined, simply because justifying thoughts are typically positive ones such as "I deserve it" and "There's nothing else in my life that I enjoy." Thoughts that justify smoking behaviors often reflect *shoulds*, "I should be entitled to have this cigarette because I've had such a terrible time."

Quite often, smokers use smoking to cope with negative emotions such as stress, low mood, or boredom, and it becomes their justification for why they deserve a cigarette. To challenge these thoughts, reflect on the real reason why you want to smoke, "If I didn't feel this way, how much would I want to smoke?" Re-evaluate the situation: "What is really going on here? Is the problem or my craving really that bad?" and "What will a cigarette do to change the situation that I am facing?" Redefine what you want to achieve from the situation (e.g., "I don't want to smoke, I want to relax") and take active steps to achieve relaxation without smoking.

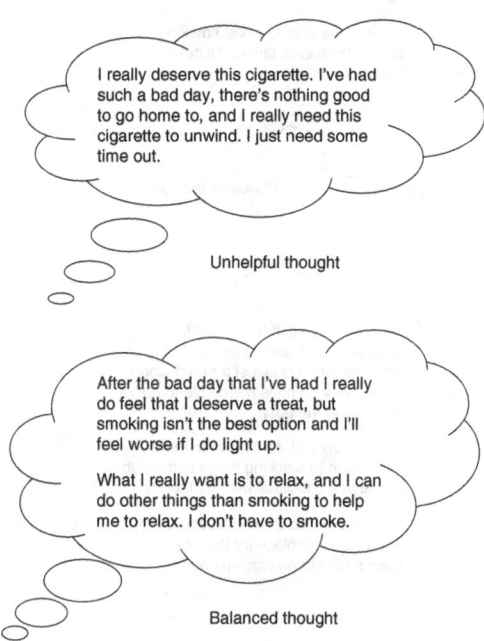

I really deserve this cigarette. I've had such a bad day, there's nothing good to go home to, and I really need this cigarette to unwind. I just need some time out.

Unhelpful thought

After the bad day that I've had I really do feel that I deserve a treat, but smoking isn't the best option and I'll feel worse if I do light up.

What I really want is to relax, and I can do other things than smoking to help me to relax. I don't have to smoke.

Balanced thought

Lapses

When lapses occur, they often prompt unhelpful thinking styles. For example, predictive thinking may be present as you think that a lapse means that you are doomed to remain smoking forever. The negative spotlight may also come into play if you think that a lapse is a sign that you have failed in your endeavor to be smoke free, while discounting all the times that you have not given in to cravings. Catastrophizing may exacerbate this belief, in that you may think that you will never become smoke free and will die of smoking-related diseases for sure.

The reality is that a lapse is a single event and it does not mean that it is inevitable that you will automatically smoke again (see also the separate handout *The change cycle: steps to becoming smoke free*). You can take active steps to change what made you more vulnerable.

It may be difficult to see this, but a lapse actually also has a positive function in that you learn about situations that make you more vulnerable to smoke. Treat a lapse as a learning experience where you learn to identify why you smoked in the first place and develop a plan to manage this high-risk situation in the future.

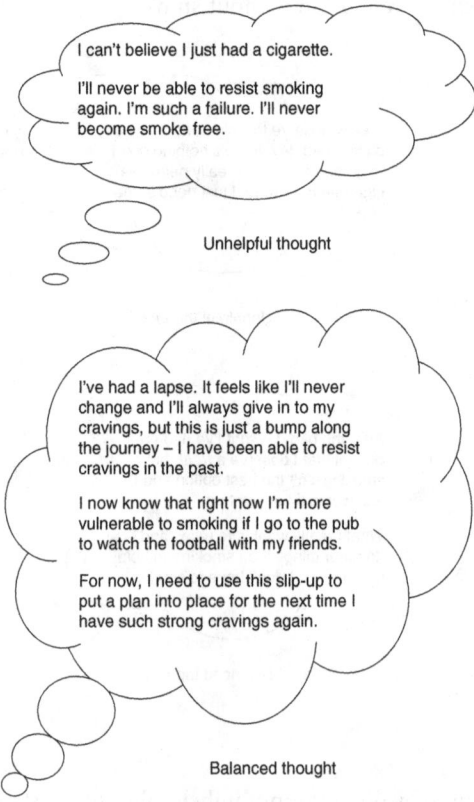

Worksheet 1 Smoking-related thoughts

Using the boxes below, list (a) thoughts that prompt your desire to smoke, (b) thoughts that justify your smoking behaviors, and (c) thoughts in response to your cravings and lapses

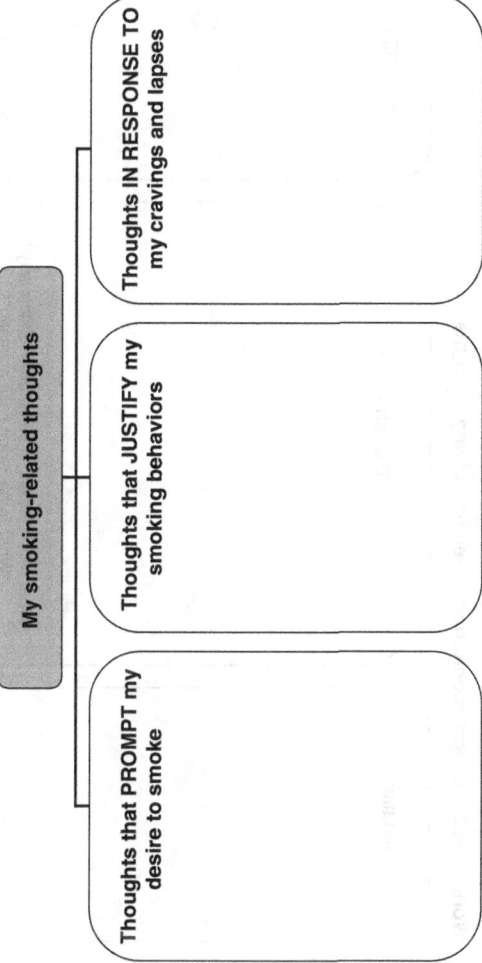

My smoking-related thoughts

Thoughts that PROMPT my desire to smoke

Thoughts that JUSTIFY my smoking behaviors

Thoughts IN RESPONSE TO my cravings and lapses

Worksheet 2 Thought monitoring sheet: identifying thoughts

Situation	Thoughts	Feelings
Where were you? What were you doing? Who else was around? When did this occur?	"What was I thinking right before I felt this way?" "What is the 'worst case scenario'?" "If this thought is true, what's so bad about it?" "What does this say about me and my abilities?" "What does this say about other people?" "What does this say about how the world works?"	How did you feel? Rate the intensity of each feeling out of 10 (10 being the most intense)

Worksheet 3 Thought monitoring sheet: example

Situation

Out at a bar for drinks on Friday night with friends after a long week at work.

A friend who is a smoker offered me a cigarette, I hesitated but ended up saying no after thinking about it for half an hour.

Where were you?
What were you doing?
Who else was around?
When did this occur?

Thoughts

I should have known that going to a bar would put me in a difficult position. I'm stupid and irresponsible.

[What does this say about you?]

→ By hesitating, it must mean that I am not committed to being smoke free.

[What does this say about the future?]

→ I'll always have to keep an eye out for vulnerable situations; I can't ever let my guard down or I will fail. I'll always struggle between wanting to approach and wanting to avoid cigarettes.

[What does this say about you?]

→ I'm weak and I will always be weak (Core belief)

"What was I thinking right before I felt this way?"
"What is the 'worst case scenario'?"
"If this thought is true, what's so bad about it?"
"What does this say about me and my abilities?"
"What does this say about other people?"
"What does this say about how the world works?"
"What does it say about the future?"

Feelings

Sad (6)
Annoyed (3)
Depressed (8)

How did you feel?

Rate the intensity of each feeling out of 10 (10 being the most intense)

Worksheet 4 Arriving at balanced thought(s): thought monitoring sheet

Situation	Thoughts	Feelings

Evidence

For:

Against:

Balanced thought(s)

Worksheet 5 Arriving at balanced thought(s): example

Situation

Out at a bar for drinks on Friday night with friends after a long week at work.

A friend who is a smoker offered me a cigarette, I hesitated but ended up saying no after thinking about it for half an hour.

Thoughts

I should have known that going to a bar would put me in a difficult position. I'm stupid and irresponsible.

→ By hesitating, it must mean that I'm not committed to being smoke free.

→ I'll always have to keep an eye out for vulnerable situations; I can't ever let my guard down or I will fail. I'll always struggle between wanting to approach and wanting to avoid cigarettes.

→ I'm weak and I will always be weak. (core belief)

Feelings

Angry at self (7)
Hopeless (5)

Evidence

For:

I do know that, right now, socializing with my friends who smoke – especially when I drink – makes me more vulnerable to smoking.

I did hesitate and had to think for half an hour about whether or not to take my friend up on the offer.

I have given in to my cravings before when the situation has been too powerful to resist.

Against:

There have been times when I've experienced very strong cravings but I have been able to resist them.

It won't always be a struggle even though it feels that way right now. I'm going through a period right now where the cravings are really intense.

Balanced thought(s)

Yes, I could have made a better decision than to go for drinks with my friend who smokes – alcohol makes me more vulnerable to smoking. I will socialize with my smoker friends in alcohol-free situations such as going to play golf or going for a coffee.

While it took me a while to say no, I *did* end up saying no. It won't always be this difficult; the cravings are just more intense right now.

Angry at self → 4
Hopeless → 2

10

Lifestyle change: on being a non-smoker

THERAPIST GUIDELINES

Aims

1 Review the rationale for focusing on lifestyle change
2 Highlight the elements in the manual that specifically contribute to the promotion of lifestyle change
3 Review the role of imagery exercises in enhancing the cognitive accessibility of a self-concept as a non-smoker
4 Review the role of motivational strategies in helping clients to shift toward a self-concept as a non-smoker
5 Use examples of imagery exercises to help clients to practice goal-directed imagery of being a non-smoker.

The rationale of lifestyle change

Becoming smoke free is not just about quitting cigarettes; it is about gaining a better life. It transforms a person from someone beholden to a debilitating addiction to someone who enjoys a healthier, cleaner, and smarter lifestyle. For many "hard-core" smokers, becoming smoke free involves taking steps into the unknown, into a world of day-to-day experiences radically different from those they had taken for granted and accepted as a part of their life as a smoker. Clients often report with amazement in their first week or two of being smoke free, how everyday experiences as a non-smoker create newfound ways of doing, sensing, or feeling. For example, one client working in an artistic profession discovered how not having one of his hands constantly preoccupied with handling a cigarette made him work more efficiently and with greater purpose; indeed, he experienced this freer way of working with his hands as if he had recovered from a physical disability that previously had restricted him to make do with only one hand. Often clients report that it feels like a mental strain has been lifted from their daily routines by not having to think every time they leave the house whether or not they have enough cigarettes with them to last them through the day, whether they have the opportunity to buy more if they run out, where they will be, and if there are places where smoking is permitted. Others plan activities that they had not even considered while still smoking. For example, a young man involved in competitive sports realized his fitness level was improving markedly and he started training for higher-level competitive events that previously would have been out of his league to even attempt. In short, becoming smoke free is not simply the absence of smoking, it transforms the ex-smoker's life in a way that changes his or her self-concept and creates new lifestyle opportunities.

Promotion of lifestyle change

Promoting lifestyle change is, therefore, an important core element of the program, as outlined in Chapter 1 of this manual. It must be remembered that being a smoker is all that most group members have known for a long time, and that many aspects of who they are as a person are associated with a smoking lifestyle. The notion of "quitting" smoking is, therefore, inevitably linked with giving up some aspects of the smokers' selves. The uncertainty of what life will be like as a non-smoker can create anxiety, which, in turn, can threaten the resolve to carry through with making the change in lifestyle. The uncertainties of these profound changes are not simply transient nuisances but are potential barriers to change to which smokers must effortfully adapt (Piasecki, 2006). Simply put, because most smokers have been habitual smokers since adolescence, they have little practical experience living as adults without smoking. Several strategies throughout the different modules in this program are designed to help clients to gain practice in shedding the routines of a smoker and replacing them with the ways a non-smoker would think, feel, and act.

Beginning with the assessment interview (Chapter 2), there is a section that elicits smoking-related background information. Specifically, two questions pertain to interests and hobbies and how these are associated with smoking. This information in useful for initiating thought processes in the smoker about how these regular activities may become altered or may be pursued in a different way once they become uncoupled from smoking. That is, the smokers are encouraged to begin imagining what their leisure activities would be like once they have commenced a smoke-free lifestyle. Similarly, the next two questions in this section of the assessment interview pertain to health and medical issues relevant to smoking. Clients can be encouraged from the start to imagine how the quality of their life would be enhanced if their health status improves as a function of becoming smoke free. For example, a client who suffered from regular sleep apnea reported after the first phase of the program a marked improvement in sleep quality after he had achieved a 50% reduction in daily cigarette intake. He reported a decrease in night-time wakening, which led to him feeling more rested in the morning; this, in turn, gave him greater energy during the day and enabled him to achieve more. This tangible change in lifestyle quality served as a strong motivator for him to take the next step of becoming smoke free and entering the maintenance phase of the program. In sum, the process of promoting lifestyle change is already initiated during the assessment phase, by identifying – and then monitoring – personal, medical, and social aspects of the client's lifestyle, which are likely to be profoundly altered by the adoption of a non-smoking lifestyle.

The use of imagery to support self-concept as non-smoker

Chapter 3 describes the first session of the program. You will recall that, in addition to initiating behavioral change strategies, one of the explicit aims of this module on starting the change process is actively to promote a shift away from a self-image as a smoker toward a self-image as a non-smoker. It was suggested that the first session should end with an imagery exercise (i.e., *From Smoke City to Fresh Hills*). The rationale for this is that through the use of imagining techniques smokers can learn to envisage life without smoking. That is, they can develop a stronger conception of themselves as a non-smoker. This new, emerging self-concept as a non-smoker can then be activated and strengthened with practice to counter and eventually replace the well-established self-concept as a smoker (Shadel & Mermelstein, 1996). In this way, the imagery exercises serve a priming function through which the, as yet novel, non-smoker self-concept is made cognitively more accessible (Shadel *et al.*, 2004). Evidence suggests that cognitively priming the abstainer self-concept increases self-efficacy and decreases craving in response to pro-vocative smoking cues (Shadel & Cervone, 2006), and a stronger self-image as a non-smoker prospectively predicts desire to quit (Lipkus *et al.*, 2005). It is for that reason that the first imagery exercise (*From Smoke City to Fresh Hills*) is introduced right at the beginning of the program, so that clients can be encouraged to start coming up with their own personalized images between sessions. Because of the strength of the existing smoker self-image, many clients initially find it difficult to imagine what a smoke-free lifestyle would be like for them. Reassure clients that this is normal, and that they will find it easier to do as they practice within and between sessions over the course of the program. An advantage of the group format is that listening to and participating in the imagery exercises of other group members often helps clients to relate the merits of this exercise to their own circumstances, and thereby create their own personalized imagery.

As mentioned in Chapter 2, the initial assessment interview included a quantitative measure of the relative strength of each client's self-concept as a smoker and a non-smoker. This provides a baseline against which the targeted shift away from a self-image as a smoker toward a self-image as a non-smoker can be monitored and evaluated at the end of the program. Ideally, at the completion of the program, the balance in the strength of the two self-concept scores will have shifted in favor of the non-smoker image. To the extent that this has not yet occurred, even if clients have remained smoke free for a period of time, those clients should be encouraged to be especially vigilant for any signs that their "old smoker selves" try to undermine the gains they have made before their new non-smoking lifestyle has become more firmly established.

Use of motivational strategies to support self-concept as non-smoker

Chapters 6 and 7 describe the motivational strategies for becoming and staying smoke free. The notion of ambivalence and the aim of developing a discrepancy between current behavior as a smoker and the desired lifestyle of a non-smoker was first introduced in Chapter 2 and then elaborated in Chapter 6 in the module on enhancing the motivation for change. The process of moving from a state of ambivalence about quitting to a state of avoidance of smoking-related behaviors can be greatly facilitated if clients simultaneously and increasingly shift their attention to what it means for them personally to be smoke free. That is, in addition to getting better at executing coping strategies that allow them to avoid smoking, they also enhance their approach coping skills, which allow them to recruit cognitive schema and behavioral routines that are congruent with the person they want to be (i.e., a non-smoker). As discussed in Chapters 6 and 7, experiencing and expressing satisfaction with progress toward the goal of being a non-smoker helps to build and maintain momentum toward achieving that goal.

Finally, it is good practice to reward clients who achieve smoke-free status at the end of the program with a certificate that highlights their achievement and marks the transition into a smoke-free lifestyle.

Tips for working with individuals

When working with an individual client, there are no opportunities to use the experiences of other group members to generate examples of anticipated lifestyle changes associated with being a non-smoker. This diminished range in diverse examples can be a disadvantage, especially

Tips (cont.)

for those individuals who have great difficulty with using their own imagination (as opposed to just *doing* something as part of the behavioral change strategies). However, the advantage of working with only one client is that one can tailor the imagery exercises very closely to the personal circumstances of this client. The sample imagery exercises provided in the *Therapist materials* of this chapter represent a range of different lifestyle changes that may occur as a function of smoking cessation. These can be used as a menu of imagery options, from which clients can select what suits them best for their personal circumstances, or from which they can derive ideas for coming up with their own personal imagery exercises.

THERAPIST MATERIALS

Six examples are given of imagery exercises to promote a self-concept as a non-smoker:
1 Going out to eat and catch a movie
2 Catching up with friends at the café
3 Enjoying a better professional image at work
4 Enjoying smoke-free family fun
5 Feeling fitter and healthier
6 Drinking in the sea breeze.

Example 1: going out to eat and catch a movie

Imagine you are smoke free now and getting ready to go out – you smell how fresh your clothes smell now – no sign of that dirty, smoky stink. The clothes feel so good on you and you're feeling excited about going out. Imagine going to a restaurant and knowing you can enjoy yourself without planning which part of the meal to interrupt to go out for a smoke or having to take a jacket because it will be cold when you go outside to smoke. You enjoy being able to stay for the whole meal and the entire conversation. You notice how much less stressful it is when you are not getting those anxious or angry looks from your friends and family that used to happen when you went out for that cigarette. After the restaurant, you look forward to going to a movie and being able to sit there and concentrate for the entire movie without continually craving a cigarette and without thinking when you can get out of there to feed that old addiction. You feel so relaxed and calm and you notice how much you are really enjoying yourself. You feel so proud of how you have been able to gain this greater enjoyment and sense of freedom by becoming smoke free.

Example 2: catching up with friends at the café

You stride across the café to meet your friends. You feel casual and relaxed, there is a spring in your step. It is a sunny day but the air is cold. As a non-smoker, you look forward to being able to remain indoors with your friends where it is warm and pleasant, rather than having to leave the conversation continually to go out for a cigarette. You feel confident that you will be able to refrain from smoking even though some of your friends are still smokers. Sitting at your table, you notice the smell of pastries wafting from the kitchen. You delight in being able to capture the fresh aroma now that your sense of smell is not so filled with smoke. You enjoying spending time at the café with your friends and you become engrossed in the conversations.

Suddenly, one of your friends noticed in surprise that you are still in the café while other friends have retreated outside for a cigarette. You are also surprised that you didn't even notice your friends had stepped outside. You glance outside to see where your friends are, and you see them huddled together against the cold, drawing on their cigarettes. You find it striking to notice that you feel so comfortable, warm, and relaxed in the café – you notice the contrast between your relaxed, non-smoking self and the awkward composure of your smoking friends, and you reflect on how you previously thought that you needed to smoke to achieve this feeling of stress relief. But now you bask in the glow of the light streaming through the window and draw in the wonderful aromas within the café. You feel so proud of your achievement in reaching a stage where you can more fully enjoy going out with friends.

Example 3: enjoying a better professional image at work

You are getting dressed for work in the morning and feeling surprisingly more energetic and strong than usual – ready to face the working day. You notice you can concentrate better and that you're feeling less anxious than usual. It's a good feeling to start each day with now. You get to work and feel relieved that you don't have to find a way to duck out for a cigarette or receive that disapproving look from your boss and colleagues. You feel proud that they notice you have improved your professional image as you smell better, seem more on top of things, concentrate better, and use your time more wisely now. You feel relief that you no longer have to spend your breaks awkwardly lingering outside the building to feed your smoking habit. Instead, you enjoy chatting in the staff room and find it a good place to unwind. You find that you are missing out on less at work now – you know more about what is going on with your work and with your work colleagues. You generally feel more on top of things, more relaxed.

Example 4: enjoying smoke free family fun

You are having a barbeque with your family and notice that you are enjoying it more than ever – the air smells fresher and you don't have to worry about what people will think or say when you have a cigarette. Your loved ones seem less on edge – more reassured that you are looking after yourself better now and that you can enjoy a longer, happier, and fuller life with them. The family plays a game of cricket after eating and you notice that you now have enough energy, not only to join in, but to chase the ball and the kids around and enthusiastically enjoy the game. Everyone is having a great time, everyone seems so relaxed and happy.

Example 5: feeling fitter and healthier

Now that you are a non-smoker, you are able to do a range of physical activities that were not that easy before. You decide to go jogging in a succulent forest after a fresh rain. As you are jogging along, you feel the soft ground cushioning your feet. You find that you can move and breathe so easily you feel like you are walking on air. While you jog, you look around at the trees passing you by. They are so vividly green, and their color is accentuated by the soft light filtering through the canopy. You drink in the warmth of the sun as it streams through the branches and gleams on your glistening body. You feel a cool breeze around you and the leaves rustling rhythmically with each swell of the breeze. You feel your lungs fill with the cool, fresh air; you smell the freshness of the forest air. Your lungs feel open and free to drink in the fresh air. You have never felt so fit and healthy.

You decide to stop and take in your scenic surroundings. You rest on a moss-covered stone bench encircled by leafy green trees. The atmosphere feels deep, still, and serene. You bathe in the warmth of the sun. You feel the breeze swell and sweep over your body from head to toe; you draw air deeply into your fresh lungs, breathing in with ease, sweeping away your tension as the wind gently moves. You feel more and more relaxed, more and more calm; you are free.

Example 6: drinking in the sea breeze

Let's imagine you are a non-smoker and have gone to a beach. You have just descended down a long flight of wooden stairs and now you find yourself standing on a stretch of the most pristine beach you have ever seen. It is wide and stretches as far as you can see in both directions. You sit down on the sand and find that it's white and smooth, warm and heavy.

You let the sand sift through your fingers and it seems almost like liquid. You lie on your stomach, finding that the warm sand instantly conforms to the shape of your body. A soft breeze touches your face. The soft sand holds you. The surf rumbles as it rises into long white crests that break towards you, then dissolve on the sand's edge. The air smells of salt and sea life, and you breathe it in deeply. There is so much air in your lungs now, they are no longer full of gunk, it's an amazing and unfamiliar feeling to feel so much fresh air in your lungs. You can feel the breeze moving over your body and moving your hair gently. You feel so happy and relaxed.

So calm and healthy and free.

References

Abrams, D. B. & Niaura, R. (2003). Planning evidence-based treatment of tobacco dependence. In D. B. Abrams, R. Niaura, R. A. Brown, *et al.* (eds.), *The Tobacco Dependence Treatment Handbook: A Guide to Best Practice*, pp. 1–26. New York: Guilford Press.

Abrams, D. B., Herzog, T. A., Emmons, K. M., & Linnan, L. (2000). Stages of change versus addiction: a replication and extension. *Nicotine and Tobacco Research*, **2**, 223–229.

Abrams, D. B., Niaura, R., Brown, R. A., *et al.* (2003). *The Tobacco Dependence Treatment Handbook: A Guide to Best Practice*. New York: Guilford Press.

Al-Shammari, K. F., Moussa, M. A., Al-Ansari, J. M., Al-Duwairy, Y. S., & Honkala, E. J. (2006). Dental patient awareness of smoking effects on oral health: comparison of smokers and non-smokers. *Journal of Dentistry*, **34**, 173–178.

Anda, R. F., Williamson, D. F., Escobedo, L. G., *et al.* (1990). Depression and the dynamics of smoking. *Journal of the American Medical Association*, **264**, 1541–1545.

Antony, M. M. & Swinson, R. P. (1998). *When Perfect Isn't Good Enough: Strategies for Coping with Perfectionism*. Oakland, CA: New Harbinger Publications.

ASH (2007, February). *Nicotine Replacement Therapy: Guidelines for Healthcare Professionals on using Nicotine Replacement Therapy for Smokers Not Yet Ready to Stop Smoking*. Woolloomooloo, Australia: ASH (www.ashaust.org.au/pdfs/NRTguide0702.pdf; accessed August 2007).

Augood, C., Duckitt, K., & Templeton, A. A. (1998). Smoking and female infertility: a systematic review and meta-analysis. *Human Reproduction*, **13**, 1532–1539.

Australian Institute of Health and Welfare (2007). *Statistics on Drug Use in Australia 2006*. [*Drug Statistics Series*, No. 18, Cat. No. PHE 80.]. Canberra: Australian Institute of Health and Welfare.

Baker, R. R. (2006). The generation of formaldehyde in cigarettes: overview and recent experiments. *Food and Chemical Toxicology*, **44**, 1799–1822.

Bauld, L., Chesterman, J., Judge, K., Pound, E., & Coleman, T. (2003). Impact of UK National Health Service smoking cessation services: variations in outcomes in England. *Tobacco Control*, **12**, 296–301.

Beck, J. B. (1995). *Cognitive Therapy: Basics and Beyond*. New York: Guilford Press.

Benowitz, N. L. (1996). Pharmacology of nicotine: addiction and therapeutics. *Annual Review of Pharmacology and Toxicology*, **36**, 597–613.

Benowitz, N. L., Jacob, P., Kozlowski, L. T., & Yu, L. (1986). Influence of smoking fewer cigarettes on exposure to tar, nicotine, and carbon monoxide. *New England Journal of Medicine*, **315**, 1310–1313.

Benowitz, N. L., Jacob, P., Bernert, J. T., et al. (2005). Carcinogen exposure during short-term switching from regular to "light" cigarettes. *Cancer Epidemiology, Biomarkers and Prevention*, **14**, 1376–1383.

Bergmann, F., Bleich, S., Wischer, S., & Paulus, W. (2002). Seizure and cardiac arrest during bupropion SR treatment. *Journal of Clinical Psychopharmacology*, **22**, 630–631.

Berlin, I. & Covey, L. S. (2006). Pre-cessation depressive mood predicts failure to quit smoking: the role of coping and personality traits. *Addiction*, **101**, 1814–1821.

Bernhard, D., Moser, C., Backovic, A., & Wick, G. (2007). Cigarette smoke: an aging accelerator? *Experimental Gerontology*, **42**, 160–165.

Bien, T. H., Miller, W. R., & Tonigan, J. S. (1993). Brief interventions for alcohol problems: a review. *Addiction*, **88**, 315–336.

Bollinger, C. T., Zellweger, J., Danielson, T., et al. (2002). Influence of long-term smoking reduction on health risk markers and quality of life. *Nicotine and Tobacco Research*, **4**, 433–439.

Brandon, T. H., Vidrine, J. I., & Litvin, E. B. (2007). Relapse and relapse prevention. *Annual Review of Clinical Psychology*, **3**, 257–284.

British American Tobacco (2006). *Australia Ingredients Report. 1 March 2005 – 1 March 2006.* Pagewood, Australia: British American Tobacco (www.aodgp.gov.au/internet/wcms/publishing.nsf/Content/health-pubhlth-strateg-drugs-tobacco-ingredients.htm; accessed March 2007).

Brown, R. A., Kahler, C. W., Niaura, R., et al. (2001). Cognitive–behavioral treatment for depression in smoking cessation. *Journal of Consulting and Clinical Psychology*, **69**, 471–480.

Buehler, R., Griffin, D., & Ross, M. (1994). Exploring the "planning fallacy": why people underestimate their task completion times. *Journal of Personality and Social Psychology*, **67**, 366–381.

Cabanac, M. & Frankham, P. (2002). Evidence that nicotine lowers the body weight set point. *Physiology and Behavior*, **76**, 539–542.

Canoy, D., Wareham, N., Luben, R., et al. (2005). Cigarette smoking and fat distribution in 21 828 British men and women: a population-based study. *Obesity Research*, **13**, 1466–1475.

Carmody, T. P. (1992). Affect regulation, nicotine addiction, and smoking cessation. *Journal of Psychoactive Drugs*, **24**, 111–112.

Catley, D., O'Connell, K. A., & Shiffman, S. (2000). Absentminded lapses during smoking cessation. *Psychology of Addictive Behaviors*, **14**, 73–76.

Chandola, T., Head, J., & Bartley, M. (2004). Socio-demographic predictors of quitting smoking: how important are household factors? *Addiction*, **99**, 770–777.

Chapman, S., Wong, W., & Smith, W. (1993). Self-exempting beliefs about smoking and health: differences between smokers and ex-smokers. *American Journal of Preventative Medicine*, **83**, 215–219.

Cinciripini, P. M., Wetter, D. W., Fouladi, R. T., et al. (2003). The effects of depressed mood on smoking cessation: medication by postcessation self-efficacy. *Journal of Consulting and Clinical Psychology*, **71**, 292–301.

Clark, M. M., Hurt, R. D., Croghan, I. T., et al. (2006). The prevalence of weight concerns in a smoking abstinence clinical trial. *Addictive Behaviors*, **31**, 1144–1152.

Cohen, S., Lichtenstein, E., Prochaska, J. O., *et al.* (1989). Debunking myths about self-quitting: evidence from 10 prospective studies of persons who attempt to quit smoking by themselves. *American Psychologist*, **44**, 1355–1365.

Cole, C. W., Hill, G. B., Farzad, E., *et al.* (1993). Cigarette smoking and peripheral arterial occlusive disease. *Surgery*, **114**, 753–757.

Compston, J. (2007). Editorial: smoking and the skeleton. *Journal of Clinical Endocrinology and Metabolism*, **92**, 428–429.

Curry, S. J. & McBride, C. M. (1994). Relapse prevention for smoking cessation: review and evaluation of concepts and interventions. *Annual Review of Public Health*, **15**, 345–366.

Curry, S. J., Ludman, E. J., & McClure, J. (2003). Self-administered treatment for smoking cessation. *Journal of Clinical Psychology*, **59**, 305–319.

Dale, L. C., Schroeder, D. R., Wolter, T. D., *et al.* (1998). Weight change after smoking cessation using variable doses of transdermal nicotine replacement. *Journal of General Internal Medicine*, **13**, 9–15.

Davis, M., Eshelman, E. R., & McKay, M. (1995). *The Relaxation and Stress Reduction Workbook*, 4th edn. Oakland, CA: New Harbinger Publications.

Department of Health (2001). *NHS Smoking Cessation Services: Services and Monitoring Guidance*. London: Department of Health.

DiClemente, C. C. (2003). *Addiction and Change: How Addiction Develops and Addicted People Recover*. New York: Guilford Press.

Dodgen, C. E. (2005). *Nicotine Dependence: Understanding and Applying the Most Effective Treatment Interventions*. Washington, DC: American Psychological Association.

Droungas, A., Ehrman, R. N., Childress, A. R., & O'Brien, C. P. (1995). Effect of smoking cues and cigarette availability on craving and smoking behaviour. *Addictive Behaviors*, **20**, 657–673.

D'Zurilla, T. J. (1988). Problem-solving therapies. In K. S. Dobson (ed.), *Handbook of Cognitive–Behavioral Therapies*. New York: Guilford Press.

Fagerström, K. (2002). The epidemiology of smoking: health consequences and benefits of cessation. *Drugs*, **62**(Suppl. 2), 1–9.

Ferguson, J., Bauld, L., Chesterman, J., & Judge, K. (2005). The English smoking treatment services: one-year outcomes. *Addiction*, **100**, 59–69.

Fergusson, D. M., Goodwin, R. D., & Harwood, L. J. (2003). Major depression and cigarette smoking: results of a 21-year longitudinal study. *Psychological Medicine*, **33**, 1357–1367.

Ferrari, J. R., Johnson, J. L., & McCown, W. G. (1995). *Procrastination and Task Avoidance. Theory, Research and Treatment*. New York: Plenum Press.

Filozof, C., Fernandez, P. M. C., & Fernandez-Cruz, A. (2004). Smoking cessation and weight gain. *Obesity Reviews*, **5**, 95–103.

Fiore, M. C., Smith, S. S., Jorenby, D. E., & Baker, T. B. (1994). The effectiveness of the nicotine patch for smoking cessation: a meta-analysis. *Journal of the American Medical Association*, **271**, 1940–1947.

Fiore, M. C., Bailey, W. C., Cohen, S. J., *et al.* (2000). *Treating Tobacco Use and Dependence: Clinical Practice Guideline*. Rockville, MD: US Department of Health and Human Services, Public Health Service.

Garvey, A. J., Bliss, R. E., Hitchcock, J. L., Heinold, J. W., & Rosner, B. (1992). Predictors of smoking relapse among self-quitters: a report from the normative aging study. *Addictive Behaviors*, **17**, 367–377.

GlaxoSmithKline (2005). *Zyban Tablets: Consumer Medicine Information.* (www.gsk. com.au/resources.ashx/prescriptionmedicinesproductschilddatadownloads/402/ File/E9228C1DD4C57F73E7675DEDFBCF4C55/CMI_Zyban.pdf; accessed August 2007).

Godtfredsen, N. S., Vestbo, J., Osler, M., & Prescott, E. (2002). Risk of hospital admission for COPD following smoking cessation and reduction: a Danish population study. *Thorax*, **57**, 967–972.

Godtfredsen, N. S., Prescott, E., & Osler, M. (2005). Effect of smoking reduction on lung cancer risk. *Journal of the American Medical Association*, **294**, 1505–1510.

Goldstein, M. G. (2003). Pharmacotherapy for smoking cessation. In D. B. Abrams, R. Niaura, R. A. Brown, et al. (eds.), *The Tobacco Dependence Treatment Handbook: A Guide to Best Practice*, pp. 230–248. New York: Guilford Press.

Greenberg, L. S. (2002). *Emotion-focused Therapy: Coaching Clients to Work Through their Feelings.* Washington, DC: American Psychological Association.

Greenberger, D. & Padesky, C. A. (1995). *Mind over Mood: Change How you Feel by Changing the Way you Think.* New York: Guilford Press.

Haas, A. L., Muñoz, R. F., Humfleet, G. L., Reus, V. I., & Hall, S. M. (2004). Influences of mood, depression history, and treatment modality on outcomes in smoking cessation. *Journal of Consulting and Clinical Psychology*, **72**, 563–570.

Haberstick, B. C., Timberlake, D., Ehringer, M. A., et al. (2007). Genes, time to first cigarette and nicotine dependence in a general population sample of young adults. *Addiction*, **102**, 655–665.

Hajek, P., Belcher, M., & Stapleton, J. (1985). Enhancing the impact of groups: an evaluation of two group formats for smokers. *British Journal of Clinical Psychology*, **24**, 289–294.

Hall, S. M., Reus, V. I., Muñoz, R. F., et al. (1998). Nortriptyline and cognitive–behavioral therapy in the treatment of cigarette smoking. *Archives of General Psychiatry*, **55**, 683–690.

Hammond, D., Fong, G. T., Cummings, K. M., & Hyland, A. (2005). Smoking topography, brand switching, and nicotine delivery: results from an in vivo study. *Cancer Epidemiology, Biomarkers and Prevention*, **14**, 1370–1375.

Health Development Agency. (2003). *Standard for Training in Smoking Cessation Treatments.* London: Health Development Agency. (www.hda-online.org.uk/ documents/smoking_cessation_treatments.pdf; accessed February 2007).

Heatherton, T. F., Kozlowski, L. T., Frecker, R. C., & Fagerström, K. (1991). The Fagerström Test for Nicotine Dependence: a revision of the Fagerström Tolerance Questionnaire. *British Journal of Addiction*, **86**, 1119–1127.

Hecht, S. S. (1999). Tobacco smoke carcinogens and lung cancer. *Journal of the National Cancer Institute*, **91**, 1194–1210.

Herzog, T. A. & Blagg, C. O. (2007). Are most precontemplators contemplating smoking cessation? Assessing the validity of the stages of change. *Health Psychology*, **26**, 222–231.

Hollon, S. D., De Rubeis, R. J., Shelton, R. C., et al. (2005). Prevention of relapse following cognitive therapy vs medications in moderate to severe depression. *Archives of General Psychiatry*, **62**, 417–422.

Hughes, J. R. (2000). Reduced smoking: an introduction and review of the evidence. *Addiction*, **95**(Suppl. 1), 3–7.

Hughes, J. R. (2002). Rigidity in measures of smoking cessation. *Addiction*, **97**, 798–799.

Hughes, J. R. (2007). Effects of abstinence from tobacco: valid symptoms and time course. *Nicotine and Tobacco Research*, **9**, 315–327.

Hughes, J. R., Keely, J., & Naud, S. (2004). Shape of the relapse curve and long-term abstinence among untreated smokers. *Addiction*, **99**, 29–38.

Hughes, J. R., Stead, L. F., & Lancaster, T. (2007). Antidepressants for smoking cessation. *Cochrane Database of Systematic Reviews* 2007, Issue 1, CD000031 (DOI: 10.1002/14651858.CD000031.pub3).

Hyland, A., Levy, D. T., Rezaishiraz, H., *et al.* (2005). Reduction in amount smoked predicts future cessation. *Psychology of Addictive Behaviors*, **19**, 221–225.

Janzon, E., Hedblad, B., Beglund, G., & Engström, G. (2004). Changes in blood pressure and body weight following smoking cessation in women. *Journal of Internal Medicine*, **255**, 266–272.

Jarvis, M. J. & Sutherland, G. (1998). Tobacco smoking. In D. W. Johnston & M. Johnston (eds.), *Health Psychology*, Vol. 8: *Comprehensive Clinical Psychology*, pp. 645–674. New York: Elsevier.

Jensen, E. X., Fusch, C. H., Jaeger, P., Peheim, E., & Horber, F. F. (1995). Impact of chronic smoking on body composition and fuel metabolism. *Journal of Clinical Endocrinology and Metabolism*, **80**, 2181–2185.

John, U., Meyer, C., Rumpf, H-J., & Hapke, U. (2004). Self-efficacy to refrain from smoking predicted by major depression and nicotine dependence. *Addictive Behaviors*, **29**, 857–866.

John, U., Hanke, M., Rumpf, H-J., & Thyrian, J. R. (2005). Smoking status, cigarettes per day, and their relationship to overweight and obesity among former and current smokers in a national adult general population sample. *International Journal of Obesity*, **29**, 1289–1294.

Jorenby, D. E., Hatsukami, D. K., Smith, S. S., *et al.* (1996). Characterization of tobacco withdrawal symptoms: transdermal nicotine reduces hunger and weight gain. *Psychopharmacology*, **128**, 130–138.

Judge, K., Bauld, L., Chesterman, J., & Ferguson, J. (2005). The English smoking treatment services: short-term outcomes. *Addiction*, **100**, 46–58.

Kahler, C. W., Brown, R. A., Ramsey, S. E., *et al.* (2002). Negative mood, depressive symptoms, and major depression after smoking cessation treated in smokers with a history of major depressive disorder. *Journal of Abnormal Psychology*, **111**, 670–675.

Kanis, J. A., Johnell, O., Oden, A., *et al.* (2005). Smoking and fracture risk: a meta-analysis. *Osteoporosis International*, **16**, 155–162.

Kapoor, D. & Jones, T. H. (2005). Smoking and hormones in health and endocrine disorders. *European Journal of Endocrinology*, **152**, 491–499.

Kelly, S. P., Thornton, J., Lyratzopoulos, G., Edwards, R., & Mitchell, P. (2004). Smoking and blindness. Strong evidence for the link, but public awareness lags. *British Medical Journal*, **6**, 537–538.

Kiel, D. P., Zhang, Y., Hannan, M. T., *et al.* (1996). The effect of smoking at different life stages on bone mineral density in elderly men and women. *Osteoporosis International*, **6**, 240–248.

King, W., Carter, S. M., Borland, R., Chapman, S., & Gray, N. (2003). The Australian tar derby: the origins and fate of a low tar harm reduction programme. *Tobacco Control*, **12**(Suppl. III), iii61–iii70.

Kinnunen, T., Doherty, K., Militello, F. S., & Garvey, A. J. (1996). Depression and smoking cessation: characteristics of depressed smokers and effects on nicotine replacement. *Journal of Consulting and Clinical Psychology*, **64**, 791–798.

Kinnunen, T., Haukkala, A., Korhonen, T., *et al.* (2006). Depression and smoking across 25 years of the normative aging study. *International Journal of Psychiatry in Medicine*, **36**, 413–426.

Koh, J. S., Kang, H., Choi, S. W., & Kim, H. O. (2002). Cigarette smoking associated with premature facial wrinkling: Image analysis of facial skin replicas. *International Journal of Dermatology*, **41**, 21–27.

Kozlowski, L. T. & O'Connor, R. J. (2002). Cigarette filter ventilation is a defective design because of misleading taste, bigger puffs, and blocked vents. *Tobacco Control*, **11**(Suppl. I), i40–i50.

Kozlowski, L. T., Giovino, G. A., Edwards, B., *et al.* (2007). Advice on using over-the-counter nicotine replacement therapy – patch, gum, or lozenge – to quit smoking. *Addictive Behaviors*, **32**, 2140–2150.

Laaksonen, M., Rahkonen, O., Martikainen, P., Karvonen, S., & Lahelma, E. (2006). Smoking and SF-36 health functioning. *Preventative Medicine*, **42**, 206–209.

Leischow, S. J. & Stitzer, M. L. (1991). Effects of smoking cessation on caloric intake and weight gain in an inpatient unit. *Psychopharmacology*, **104**, 522–526.

Lerman, C., Niaura, R., Collins, B. N., *et al.* (2004). Effect of bupropion on depression symptoms in a smoking cessation clinical trial. *Psychology of Addictive Behaviors*, **18**, 362–366.

Levine, M. D., Perkins, K. A., & Marcus, M. D. (2001). The characteristics of women smokers concerned about postcessation weight gain. *Addictive Behaviors*, **26**, 749–756.

Lipkus, I. M., Pollak, K. I., McBride, C. M., *et al.* (2005). Assessing attitudinal ambivalence towards smoking and its association with desire to quit among teen smokers. *Psychology and Health*, **20**, 373–387.

Lissner, L., Bengtsson, C., Lapidus, L., & Björklund, C. (1992). Smoking initiation and cessation in relation to body fat distribution based on data from a study of Swedish women. *American Journal of Public Health*, **82**, 273–275.

Marlatt, G. A. & Gordon, J. R. (1985). *Relapse Prevention: Maintenance Strategies in the Treatment of Addictive Behaviors*. New York: Guilford Press.

McEwen, A., Hajek, P., McRobbie, H., & West, R. (2006). *Manual of Smoking Cessation: A Guide for Counsellors and Practitioners*. Oxford, UK: Blackwell.

Miller, M. & Wood, L. (2002). *Smoking Cessation Interventions: Review of Evidence and Implications for Best Practice in Health Care Settings*. Canberra, Australia: Commonwealth Department of Health and Ageing.

Miller, W. R. (1995). Increasing motivation for change. In R. K. Hester & W. R. Miller (eds.), *Handbook of Alcoholism Treatment Approaches: Effective Alternatives*, 2nd edn, pp. 89–104. Boston, MA: Allyn and Bacon.

Miller, W. R. (1998). Enhancing motivation for change. In W. R. Miller & N. Hester (eds.), *Treating Addictive Behaviors*, 2nd edn, pp. 121–132. New York: Plenum Press.

Miller, W. R. & Hester, N. (eds.). (1998). *Treating Addictive Behaviors*, 2nd edn. New York: Plenum Press.

Miller, W. R. & Rollnick, S. (2002). *Motivational Interviewing: Preparing People for Change*, 2nd edn. New York: Guilford Press.

Mitchell, P., Chapman, S., & Smith, W. (1999). Smoking is a major cause of blindness. *Medical Journal of Australia*, **171**, 173–174.

Mooney, M. E. & Hatsukami, D. K. (2001). Combined treatments for smoking cessation. In M. T. Sammons & N. B. Schmidt (eds.), *Combined Treatments for Mental Disorders: A Guide to Psychological and Pharmacological Interventions*. Washington, DC: American Psychological Association.

Morrell, H. E. R. & Cohen, L. M. (2006). Cigarette smoking, anxiety, and depression. *Journal of Psychopathology and Behavioral Assessment*, **28**, 283–297.

Morrison, N. (2002). Group cognitive therapy: treatment of choice or sub-optimal option? *Behavioural and Cognitive Psychotherapy*, **29**, 311–332.

Munafò, M., Murphy, M., Whiteman, D., & Hey, K. (2002). Does cigarette smoking increase time to conception? *Journal of Biosocial Science*, **34**, 65–73.

National Institute for Clinical Excellence (2002). *Guidance on the Use of Nicotine Replacement Therapy (NRT) and Bupropion for Smoking Cessation*. London: National Institute for Clinical Excellence.

Niaura, R. & Shadel, W. G. (2003). Assessment to inform smoking cessation treatment. In D. B. Abrams, R. Niaura, R. A. Brown, *et al.* (eds.), *The Tobacco Dependence Treatment Handbook*, pp. 27–72. New York: Guilford Press.

Norcross, J. C., Mrykalo, M. S., & Blagys, M. D. (2002). Auld lang syne: success predictors, change processes, and self-reported outcomes of New Year's resolvers and nonresolvers. *Journal of Clinical Psychology*, **58**, 397–405.

O'Brien, C. P. (1997). Recent developments in the pharmacotherapy of substance abuse. In G. A. Marlatt & G. R. VandenBos (eds.), *Addictive Behaviours*. Washington, DC: American Psychological Society.

Ockene, I. S. & Miller, N. H. (1997). Cigarette smoking, cardiovascular disease, and stroke. *Circulation*, **96**, 3243–3247.

O'Hara, P., Connett, J. E., Lee, W. W., *et al.* (1998). Early and late weight gain following smoking cessation in the lung health study. *American Journal of Epidemiology*, **148**, 821–830.

Padesky, C. A. & Greenberger, D. (1995). *Clinician's Guide to Mind Over Mood*. New York: Guilford Press.

Page, A. C. & Stritzke, W. G. K. (2006). *Clinical Psychology for Trainees: Foundations of Science-informed Practice*. Cambridge, UK: Cambridge University Press.

Parrott, A. C. (1999). Does cigarette smoking cause stress? *American Psychologist*, **54**, 817–820.

Paykel, E. S., Scott, J., Teasdale, J. D., *et al.* (1999). Prevention of relapse in residual depression by cognitive therapy. A controlled trial. *Archives of General Psychiatry*, **56**, 829–835.

Petitjean, A., Mac-Mary, S., Sainthillier, J.-M., Muret, P., & Humbert, P. (2006). Effects of cigarette smoking on the skin of women. *Journal of Dermatological Science*, **42**, 259–261.

Philip Morris Ltd. (2006). *Australian Ingredients Report. 1 March 2005 – 1 March 2006*. Moorabbin, Australia: Philip Morris Ltd. (www.aodgp.gov.au/internet/wcms/publishing.nsf/Content/health-pubhlth-strateg-drugs-tobacco-ingredients.htm; accessed March 2007).

Piasecki, T. M. (2006). Relapse to smoking. *Clinical Psychology Review*, **26**, 196–215.

Prochaska, J. O., DiClemente, C. C., & Norcross, J. C. (1992). In search of how people change: applications to addictive behaviors. *American Psychologist*, **47**, 1102–1114.

Psinger, C. & Jorgensen, T. (2007). Weight concerns and smoking in a general population: the Inter99 study. *Preventative Medicine*, **44**, 283–289.

Raw, M., McNeill, A., & West, R. (1998). Smoking cessation guidelines for health professionals: A guide to effective smoking cessation interventions for the health care system. *Thorax*, **53**(Suppl. 5), 1–19.

Rose, J. E. & Behm, F. M. (2004). Effects of low nicotine content cigarettes on smoke intake. *Nicotine and Tobacco Research*, **6**, 309–319.

Rothblum, E., Solomon, L., & Murakami, J. (2003). Affective, cognitive and behavioral differences between high and low procrastinators. *Journal of Counselling Psychology*, **33**, 387–394.

Rothman, A. J. (2000). Toward a theory-based analysis of behavioral maintenance. *Health Psychology*, **19**(Suppl. 1), 64–69.

Schafer, W. (1992). *Stress Management for Wellness*, 2nd edn. Fort Worth, TX: Harcourt Brace for Jovanovich College Publishers.

Scherer, G. (1999). Smoking behaviour and compensation: a review of the literature. *Psychopharmacology*, **145**, 1–20.

Schlaud, M., Kleemann, W. J., Poets, C. F., & Sens, B. (1996). Smoking during pregnancy and poor antenatal care: two major preventable risk factors for sudden infant death syndrome. *International Journal of Epidemiology*, **25**, 959–965.

Sepinwall, D. & Borrelli, B. (2004). Older, medically ill smokers are concerned about weight gain after quitting smoking. *Addictive Behaviors*, **29**, 1809–1819.

Shadel, W. G. & Cervone, D. (2006). Evaluating social–cognitive mechanisms that regulate self-efficacy in response to provocative smoking cues: an experimental investigation. *Psychology of Addictive Behaviors*, **20**, 91–96.

Shadel, W. G. & Mermelstein, R. (1996). Individual differences in self-concept among smokers attempting to quit: validation and predictive utility of measures of the smoker self-concept and abstainer self-concept. *Annals of Behavioral Medicine*, **18**, 151–156.

Shadel, W. G., Cervone, D., Niaura, R., & Abrams, D. B. (2004). Developing an integrative social–cognitive strategy for personality assessment at the level of the individual: an illustration with regular cigarette smokers. *Journal of Research in Personality*, **38**, 394–419.

Shah, T., Sullivan, K., & Carter, J. (2006). Sudden infant death syndrome and reported maternal smoking during pregnancy. *American Journal of Public Health*, **96**, 1757–1759.

Shiffman, S., Patten, C., Gwaltney, C., et al. (2006). Natural history of nicotine withdrawal. *Addiction*, **101**, 1822–1832.

Shiffrin, S. & Waters, A. J. (2004). Negative affect and smoking lapses: A prospective analysis. *Journal of Consulting and Clinical Psychology*, **72**, 92–201.

Silagy, C., Lancaster, T., Stead, L., Mant, D., & Fowler, G. (2004). Nicotine replacement therapy for smoking cessation. *Cochrane Database of Systematic Reviews*, Issue 3, CD000146 (DOI: 10.1002/14651858.CD000146.pub2).

Spring, B., Doran, N., Pagoto, S., et al. (2007). Fluoxetine, smoking, and history of major depression: a randomized controlled trial. *Journal of Consulting and Clinical Psychology*, **75**, 85–94.

Strasser, A. A., Lerman, C., Sanborn, P. M., Pickworth, W. B., & Feldman, E. A. (2007). New lower nicotine cigarettes can produce compensatory smoking and increased carbon monoxide exposure. *Drug and Alcohol Dependence*, **86**, 294–300.

Stritzke, W. G. K., Breiner, M. J., Curtin, J. J., & Lang, A. R. (2004). Assessment of substance cue reactivity: advances in reliability, specificity, and validity. *Psychology of Addictive Behaviors*, **18**, 148–159.

Stritzke, W. G. K., McEvoy, P. M., Wheat, L. R., Dyer, K. R., & French, D. J. (2007). The yin and yang of indulgence and restraint: the ambivalence model of craving. In P. W. O'Neal (ed.), *Motivation of Health Behavior*, pp. 31–47. Hauppauge, NY: Nova Science.

Taylor, A. H., Ussher, M. H., & Faulkner, G. (2007). The acute effects of exercise on cigarette cravings, withdrawal symptoms, affect and smoking behaviour: a systematic review. *Addiction*, **102**, 534–543.

Taylor, D. H., Hasselblad, V., Henley, S. J., Thun, M. J., & Sloan, F. A. (2002). Benefits of smoking cessation for longevity. *American Journal of Public Health*, **92**, 990–996.

Tengs, T. O. & Osgood, N. D. (2001). The link between smoking and impotence: two decades of evidence. *Preventative Medicine*, **32**, 447–452.

Tiffany, S. T. (1990). A cognitive model of drug urges and drug-use behaviour: role of automatic and nonautomatic processes. *Psychological Review*, **97**, 147–168.

Trummer, H., Habermann, H., Haas, J., & Pummer, K. (2002). The impact of cigarette smoking on human semen parameters and hormones. *Human Reproduction*, **17**, 1554–1559.

Tsoh, J. Y. & Hall, S. M. (2004). Depression and smoking: from the transtheoretical model of change perspective. *Addictive Behaviors*, **29**, 801–805.

Tsoh, J. Y., McClure, J. B., Skaar, K. L., *et al.* (1997). Smoking cessation 2: components of effective intervention. *Behavioral Medicine*, **23**, 15–27.

Tziomalos, K. & Charsoulis, F. (2004). Endocrine effects of tobacco smoking. *Clinical Endocrinology*, **61**, 664–674.

US Department of Health and Human Services. (1991). *The Health Benefits of Smoking Cessation*. [*DHHS Publication* (CDC) 90-8416]. Rockville, MD: US Department of Health and Human Services. Public Health Service. Centre for Disease Control. Centre for Chronic Disease Prevention and Health Promotion. Office on Smoking and Health (http://profiles.nlm.nih.gov/NN/B/B/C/T/_/nnbbct.pdf; accessed December 2007).

US Department of Health and Human Services. (2004). *The Health Consequences of Smoking: What It Means to You*. Rockville, MD: US Department of Health and Human Services, Centers for Disease Control and Prevention, National Center for Chronic Disease Prevention and Health Promotion, Office on Smoking and Health (www.cdc.gov/tobacco/data_statistics/sgr/sgr_2004/00_pdfs/SGR2004_Whatitmeanstoyou.pdf; accessed December 2007).

Vineis, P., Alavanja, M., Buffler, P., *et al.* (2004). Tobacco and cancer: recent epidemiological evidence. *Journal of the National Cancer Institute*, **96**, 99–106.

Wack, J. T. & Rodin, J. (1982). Smoking and its effects on body weight and the systems of caloric regulation. *American Journal of Clinical Nutrition*, **35**, 366–380.

Walsh, P. M., Carrillo, P., Flores, G., *et al.* (2007). Effects of partner smoking status and gender on long term abstinence rates of patients receiving smoking cessation treatment. *Addictive Behaviors*, **32**, 128–136.

Ward, K. D. & Klesges, R. C. (2001). A meta-analysis of the effects of cigarette smoking on bone mineral density. *Calcified Tissue International*, **68**, 259–270.

Wennike, P., Danielsson, T., Landfeldt, B., Westin, Å., & Tønnesen, P. (2003). Smoking reduction promotes smoking cessation: results from a double blind, randomized, placebo-controlled trial of nicotine gum with 2-year follow-up. *Addiction*, **98**, 1395–1402.

West, R. (2005). *Assessing Smoking Cessation Performance in NHS Stop Smoking Services: The Russell Standard (Clinical)*. London: Smoking Cessation Services Research Network (www.scsrn.org/clinical_tools/russell_standard_clinical.pdf; accessed April 2007).

West, R. (2007). The clinical significance of "small" effects of smoking cessation treatments. *Addiction*, **102**, 506–509.

West, R. & Shiffman, S. (2004). *Smoking Cessation. Fast Facts: Indispensable Guides to Clinical Practice*. Oxford: Health Press.

West, R., McNeill, A., & Raw, M. (2000). Smoking cessation guidelines for health professionals: an update. *Thorax*, **55**, 987–999.

Wilhelm, K., Wedgewood, L., Niven, H., & Kay-Lambkin, F. (2006). Smoking cessation and depression: current knowledge and future directions. *Drug and Alcohol Review*, **25**, 97–107.

Wong, P. K. K., Christie, J. J., & Wark, J. D. (2007). The effects of smoking on bone health. *Clinical Science*, **113**, 233–241.

Woody, S. R., Detweiler-Bedell, J., Teachman, B. A., & O'Hearn, T. (2003). *Treatment Planning in Psychotherapy: Taking the Guesswork out of Clinical Care*. New York: Guilford Press.

Yzer, M. & van den Putte, B. (2006). Understanding smoking cessation: the role of smokers' quit history. *Psychology of Addictive Behaviors*, **20**, 356–361.

Zhu, S., Sun, J., Hawkins, S., Pierce, J., & Cummins, S. (2003). A population study of low-rate smokers: quitting history and instability over time. *Health Psychology*, **22**, 245–252.

Index

Printed in the United States
by Baker & Taylor Publisher Services

Printed in the United States
by Baker & Taylor Publisher Services